*Lamanna*

# PRIMARY CARE AND PUBLIC HEALTH
## Exploring Integration to Improve Population Health

Committee on Integrating Primary Care and Public Health

Board on Population Health and Public Health Practice

## INSTITUTE OF MEDICINE
*OF THE NATIONAL ACADEMIES*

D1113234

THE NATIONAL ACADEMIES PRESS
Washington, D.C.
**www.nap.edu**

THE NATIONAL ACADEMIES PRESS     500 Fifth Street, NW     Washington, DC 20001

NOTICE: The project that is the subject of this report was approved by the Governing Board of the National Research Council, whose members are drawn from the councils of the National Academy of Sciences, the National Academy of Engineering, and the Institute of Medicine. The members of the committee responsible for the report were chosen for their special competences and with regard for appropriate balance.

This study was supported by Contract Nos. 200-2005-13434 and HHSH250200976014I between the National Academy of Sciences, Centers for Disease Control and Prevention and the Health Resources and Services Administration and funding from the United Health Foundation. Any opinions, findings, conclusions, or recommendations expressed in this publication are those of the author(s) and do not necessarily reflect the view of the organizations or agencies that provided support for this project.

International Standard Book Number-13:   978-0-309-25520-2
International Standard Book Number-10:   0-309-25520-1

Additional copies of this report are available from the National Academies Press, 500 Fifth Street, NW, Keck 360, Washington, DC 20001; (800) 624-6242 or (202) 334-3313; http://www.nap.edu.

For more information about the Institute of Medicine, visit the IOM home page at: www.iom.edu.

The serpent has been a symbol of long life, healing, and knowledge among almost all cultures and religions since the beginning of recorded history. The serpent adopted as a logotype by the Institute of Medicine is a relief carving from ancient Greece, now held by the Staatliche Museen in Berlin.

Cover design by LeAnn Locher.

Suggested citation: IOM (Institute of Medicine). 2012. *Primary Care and Public Health: Exploring Integration to Improve Population Health*. Washington, DC: The National Academies Press.

*"Knowing is not enough; we must apply.*
*Willing is not enough; we must do."*
—Goethe

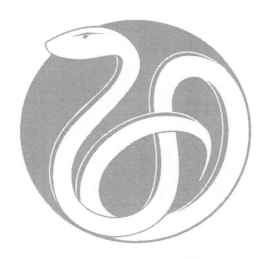

# INSTITUTE OF MEDICINE
## *OF THE NATIONAL ACADEMIES*

**Advising the Nation. Improving Health.**

# THE NATIONAL ACADEMIES
*Advisers to the Nation on Science, Engineering, and Medicine*

The **National Academy of Sciences** is a private, nonprofit, self-perpetuating society of distinguished scholars engaged in scientific and engineering research, dedicated to the furtherance of science and technology and to their use for the general welfare. Upon the authority of the charter granted to it by the Congress in 1863, the Academy has a mandate that requires it to advise the federal government on scientific and technical matters. Dr. Ralph J. Cicerone is president of the National Academy of Sciences.

The **National Academy of Engineering** was established in 1964, under the charter of the National Academy of Sciences, as a parallel organization of outstanding engineers. It is autonomous in its administration and in the selection of its members, sharing with the National Academy of Sciences the responsibility for advising the federal government. The National Academy of Engineering also sponsors engineering programs aimed at meeting national needs, encourages education and research, and recognizes the superior achievements of engineers. Dr. Charles M. Vest is president of the National Academy of Engineering.

The **Institute of Medicine** was established in 1970 by the National Academy of Sciences to secure the services of eminent members of appropriate professions in the examination of policy matters pertaining to the health of the public. The Institute acts under the responsibility given to the National Academy of Sciences by its congressional charter to be an adviser to the federal government and, upon its own initiative, to identify issues of medical care, research, and education. Dr. Harvey V. Fineberg is president of the Institute of Medicine.

The **National Research Council** was organized by the National Academy of Sciences in 1916 to associate the broad community of science and technology with the Academy's purposes of furthering knowledge and advising the federal government. Functioning in accordance with general policies determined by the Academy, the Council has become the principal operating agency of both the National Academy of Sciences and the National Academy of Engineering in providing services to the government, the public, and the scientific and engineering communities. The Council is administered jointly by both Academies and the Institute of Medicine. Dr. Ralph J. Cicerone and Dr. Charles M. Vest are chair and vice chair, respectively, of the National Research Council.

**www.nationalacademies.org**

# COMMITTEE ON INTEGRATING PRIMARY CARE AND PUBLIC HEALTH

**MARY WELLIK,** Community Health Services Administrator (Retired), Olmsted County Public Health Services, Rochester, MN
**WINSTON F. WONG,** Medical Director, Community Benefit Disparities Improvement and Quality Initiatives, National Program Office, Kaiser Permanente, Oakland, CA

*Consultants*

**SARA ROSENBAUM,** George Washington University School of Public Health and Health Services, Washington, DC
**PHILIP SLOANE,** University of North Carolina at Chapel Hill
**KATRINA DONAHUE,** University of North Carolina at Chapel Hill
**FEDERAL FUNDS INFORMATION FOR STATES,** Washington, DC
**RONA BRIERE,** Briere Associates, Inc., Felton, PA

*Staff*

**MONICA N. FEIT,** Study Director
**JOSHUA JOSEPH,** Associate Program Officer
**TREVONNE WALFORD,** Research Associate
**ANDRES GAVIRIA,** Senior Program Assistant (from August 2011)
**KATHLEEN McGRAW-SHEPHERD,** Senior Program Assistant (until August 2011)
**RACHEL MIRIANI,** Intern, Summer 2011
**ROSE MARIE MARTINEZ,** Director, Board on Population Health and Public Health Practice

# Reviewers

This report has been reviewed in draft form by individuals chosen for their diverse perspectives and technical expertise, in accordance with procedures approved by the National Research Council's Report Review Committee. The purpose of this independent review is to provide candid and critical comments that will assist the institution in making its published report as sound as possible and to ensure that the report meets institutional standards for objectivity, evidence, and responsiveness to the study charge. The review comments and draft manuscript remain confidential to protect the integrity of the deliberative process. We wish to thank the following individuals for their review of this report:

**Bobbie Berkowitz,** Columbia University School of Nursing and
     Columbia University Medical Center
**Kurtis Elward,** Family Medicine of Albemarle
**Barbara Ferrer,** Boston Public Health Commission
**Michael Katz,** March of Dimes Foundation
**Mitch Katz,** Los Angeles County Department of Health Services
**Paula Lantz,** The George Washington University
**David O. Meltzer,** University of Chicago
**James W. Mold,** University of Oklahoma Health Sciences Center
**Joshua M. Sharfstein,** Maryland Department of Health and Mental
     Hygiene
**William Welton,** University of Washington
**Steven H. Woolf,** Virginia Commonwealth University Center on
     Human Needs

Although the reviewers listed above have provided many constructive comments and suggestions, they were not asked to endorse the report's conclusions or recommendations, nor did they see the final draft of the report before its release. The review of this report was overseen by **Susan J. Curry,** The University of Iowa, and **Mark R. Cullen,** Stanford University. Appointed by the National Research Council and Institute of Medicine, they were responsible for making certain that an independent examination of this report was carried out in accordance with institutional procedures and that all review comments were carefully considered. Responsibility for the final content of this report rests entirely with the authoring committee and the institution.

# Acknowledgments

The Institute of Medicine (IOM) Committee on the Integration of Primary Care and Public Health would like to express its sincere gratitude to everyone who assisted with this report.

This work would not have been possible without the support of our sponsors. The committee would like to thank the Health Resources and Services Administration (HRSA), the Centers for Disease Control and Prevention (CDC), and the United Health Foundation for their generous sponsorship. We appreciate the time taken by Mary Wakefield, Ph.D., R.N., administrator of HRSA; Sarah Linde-Feucht, M.D., chief public health officer, HRSA; Judith Monroe, M.D., director, Office for State, Tribal, Local and Territorial Support, CDC; Chesley Richards, M.D., M.P.H., FACP, director, Office of Prevention through Healthcare, Office of the Associate Director for Policy, CDC; and Reed Tuckson, M.D., FACP, executive vice president and chief of medical affairs, UnitedHealth Group for meeting with the committee to clarify its charge. In addition, we would like to acknowledge the following staff for their assistance throughout the study:

*HRSA*

Natasha Coulouris, M.P.H.
Matthew Burke, M.D.
Chris DeGraw, M.D., M.P.H.
Seiji Hayashi, M.D., M.P.H.
Suzanne Heurtin-Roberts, Ph.D., M.S.W.
Michele Lawler, M.S., R.D.

Beverly Wright, C.N.M., M.S.N., M.P.H.
Audrey Yowell, Ph.D., M.S.S.S.

### CDC

Paula Staley, M.P.A., R.N.
Wanda Barfield, M.D., M.P.H., FAAP
Peter Briss, M.D., M.P.H.
Lydia Ogden, Ph.D., M.P.P., M.A.
Marcus Plescia, M.D., M.P.H.
Michael Schooley, M.P.H.

### United Health Foundation

Shelly Espinosa, M.P.H.

The committee would like to acknowledge and thank the many individuals who presented to the committee and provided insight on various topics throughout the study. These individuals include many of the staff listed above as well as those listed below.

Charlie Alfero, M.A. (Hidalgo Medical Service)
Alina Alonso, M.D. (Palm Beach County Health Department, Florida Department of Health)
Katherine Brieger, M.A., R.D., CDE (Hudson River Health Care)
Helen Darling, M.A. (National Business Group on Health)
Ralph Fuccillo, M.A. (DentaQuest Foundation)
M. Chris Gibbons, M.D., M.P.H. (Johns Hopkins Urban Health Institute)
Ben Gramling (Sixteenth Street Community Health Center)
Jean Johnson, Ph.D., FAAN (The George Washington University School of Nursing)
David B. Nash, M.D., M.B.A., FACP (Jefferson School of Population Health)
Robert Resendes, M.B.A. (Yavapai County Community Health Services)
Barbara Safriet, J.D., L.L.M. (Lewis & Clark Law School)
Ellen-Marie Whelan, Ph.D., N.P., R.N. (Center for Medicare & Medicaid Services Innovation Center)
Steven Woolf, M.D., M.P.H. (Virginia Commonwealth University Center on Human Needs)

Finally, the committee would like to recognize the consultants who aided in the creation of the report, Sara Rosenbaum, Philip Sloane, Katrina Donahue, and the Federal Funds Information for States organization. Their efforts proved invaluable to the committee. The committee is also grateful to Rona Briere and Alisa Decatur of Briere and Associates, Inc., for their assistance in editing the report and to LeAnn Locher for her work in creating the cover and the design elements throughout the report.

# Preface

In 2010, the Institute of Medicine (IOM) was asked by the Centers for Disease Control and Prevention (CDC) and the Health Resources and Services Administration (HRSA) to convene a committee to study and prepare a report providing recommendations on how they, as national agencies, could work collectively to improve health through the integration of primary care and public health. The CDC and HRSA sponsorship was reinforced by support from the United Health Foundation. To conduct this study, the IOM formed the Committee on Integrating Primary Care and Public Health.

This effort is not the first, nor will it likely be the last, to explore how these two sectors can complement each other and align their resources to improve population health. At the same time, the committee had a strong appreciation for the unique contributions, accountabilities, and perspectives of both sectors and respected those attributes in proposing opportunities for expanded collaboration.

Several factors contribute to the timeliness of this report with respect to both the demand for and an environment conducive to meaningful progress. Key among these factors is the sponsorship of this effort by organizations with national perspective and influence that are motivated to find ways to leverage their resources in a more collaborative manner. All of the study's sponsors are increasingly focused on various aspects of population health, including maternal and child health; cancer prevention; and management of noncommunicable chronic diseases, such as obesity, diabetes, and heart disease. The science of management of these conditions is continually being refined, and innovations in population-focused care services are rapidly evolving. The accelerating use of health information technologies has the potential to extend access to high-quality, evidence-based care to all members of the population. Finally, investments under the American Recovery and Reinvestment Act, together with the passage and ongoing implementation of the Patient Protection and Affordable Care Act, support widespread and increasingly consequential change in how health care is delivered to and accessed by Americans.

In addressing its charge and producing this report, the committee sought to find the right balance between a grand vision of enhanced population health and the need to offer actionable recommendations for the sponsoring organizations. The committee appreciated the sponsors' leadership and commitment to pursuing this endeavor, as well as the thoughtful and enthusiastic participation of many agency staff members in testimony on and discussion of existing services and considerations for future change. The committee acknowledges the complexity and challenges of effecting large-scale change in organizations with rich histories, traditions of advocacy and leadership at the agency level, and ongoing responsibilities for traditional activities.

The committee also had the opportunity to examine and learn from many initiatives designed to better align and integrate the targeted services at the local and community levels. This experience highlighted a key challenge: across the nation, most efforts to integrate care delivery and improvement in primary care and public health are locally led and defined, and there are very few examples of successful integration on a larger scale. Consequently, the committee sought to draw key principles from these local and community successes and to propose how those principles might guide actions at the national level.

Overall, the committee sought to provide strategic and practical guidance that could be implemented with anticipated resources and leadership commitment while fully leveraging emerging opportunities in the knowledge, policy, funding, and information technology environments. This guidance is built on the committee's conclusions with respect to how population health can be improved by implementing and expanding integration *now*, with the belief and intent that the momentum achievable through these changes can catalyze future progress toward a truly transformed, robust, and equitable population health system.

Paul J. Wallace, *Chair*
Committee on Integrating Primary Care and Public Health

# Contents

# Boxes, Figures, and Tables

## BOXES

## FIGURES

*xvii*

## TABLES

# Acronyms and Abbreviations

| | |
|---|---|
| ABCS | aspirin use, blood pressure control, cholesterol management, and smoking cessation |
| ACA | Patient Protection and Affordable Care Act |
| ACF | Administration for Children and Families |
| ACO | accountable care organization |
| AHRQ | Agency for Healthcare Research and Quality |
| ARRA | American Recovery and Reinvestment Act |
| | |
| CBO | Congressional Budget Office |
| CCNC | Community Care of North Carolina |
| CDC | Centers for Disease Control and Prevention |
| CHIP | Children's Health Insurance Program |
| CMMI | CMS Innovation Center |
| CMS | Centers for Medicare & Medicaid Services |
| COPC | community-oriented primary care |
| | |
| DHI | Durham Health Innovations |
| | |
| EIS | Epidemic Intelligence Service |
| | |
| FOBT | fecal occult blood test |
| FQHC | federally qualified health center |
| | |
| HERO | Health Extension Rural Office |
| HHS | Department of Health and Human Services |

| | |
|---|---|
| HIT | health information technology |
| HITECH | Health Information Technology for Economic and Clinical Health (Act) |
| HPRN | High Plains Research Network |
| HRSA | Health Resources and Services Administration |
| | |
| INPC | Indiana Network for Patient Care |
| IOM | Institute of Medicine |
| IRS | Internal Revenue Service |
| | |
| MCH | maternal and child health |
| | |
| NACCHO | National Association of County and City Health Officials |
| NAS | National Academy of Sciences |
| NHSC | National Health Service Corps |
| NIH | National Institutes of Health |
| NYC DOHMH | New York City Department of Health and Mental Hygiene |
| | |
| PCEP | Primary Care Extension Program |
| PRAMS | Pregnancy Risk Assessment Monitoring System |
| PPS | Prospective Payment System |
| | |
| REACH | Regional Electronic Adoption Center for Health |
| | |
| SPARC | Sickness Prevention Achieved through Regional Collaboration |
| SSBG | Social Services Block Grant |
| | |
| UDS | Uniform Data System |
| | |
| WHO | World Health Organization |

# Summary

Ensuring that members of society are healthy and reaching their full potential requires the prevention of disease and injury; the promotion of health and well-being; the assurance of conditions in which people can be healthy; and the provision of timely, effective, and coordinated health care. A wide array of actors across the United States—including those in both primary care[1] and public health—contribute to one or more of these elements, but their work is often carried out in relative isolation. Achieving substantial and lasting improvements in population health[2] will require a concerted effort from all of these entities, aligned with a common goal. The integration of primary care and public health could enhance the capacity of both sectors to carry out their respective missions and link with other stakeholders to catalyze a collaborative, intersectoral movement toward improved population health.

In recognition of this potential, the Health Resources and Services Administration (HRSA) and the Centers for Disease Control and Prevention (CDC) requested that the Institute of Medicine (IOM) convene a committee of experts to examine the integration of primary care and public health. The 17-member Committee on Integrating Primary Care and Public Health comprises experts in primary health care, state and local public health, ser-

---

[1]The committee recognizes that mental health is an inextricable part of primary care. When primary care is discussed in this report, the committee means it to be inclusive of mental health.

[2]When discussing the term "population health," the committee chose to adopt Kindig and Stoddart's definition (2003, p. 381): "the health outcomes of a group of individuals, including the distribution of such outcomes within the group."

*1*

vice integration, health disparities, health information technology, health care finance, health care policy, public health law, workforce education and training, organizational management, and child health. The committee was charged to:

- Identify the best examples of effective public health and primary care integration and the factors that promote and sustain these efforts. These examples were to illustrate shared accountability; workforce integration; collaborative governance, financing, and care coordination; and the effective use of information technology to promote integration and achieve high-quality primary care and public health.
- Examine ways by which HRSA and CDC can use provisions of the Patient Protection and Affordable Care Act (ACA) to promote the integration of primary care and public health.
- Discuss how HRSA-supported primary care systems and state and local public health departments can effectively integrate and coordinate to improve efforts directed at cardiovascular disease prevention, as well as other issues relevant to health disparities or specific populations, such as maternal and child health and colorectal cancer screening, and describe actions HRSA and CDC should take to promote these changes.

Funding for this study was provided by HRSA, CDC, and the United Health Foundation.

In conducting the study, the committee held five formal meetings, as well as three subgroup meetings, and used a variety of sources: the published literature, discussions with HRSA and CDC, presentations from practitioners, and commissioned papers. In drawing on these sources, the committee developed a list of key principles for the integration of primary care and public health, which are outlined below and discussed in detail in Chapter 2. These principles were used as a guiding framework in presenting examples of successful integration, identifying opportunities for interagency collaboration, and formulating the recommendations presented in this report.

## KEY TERMS

### Primary Care

The committee adopted an earlier IOM definition of primary care: "the provision of integrated, accessible health care services by clinicians who are accountable for addressing a large majority of personal health care needs, developing a sustained partnership with patients, and practicing in the context of family and community" (IOM, 1996, p. 1). Primary care in the United States is delivered through both private providers and those supported by government agencies, such as the Veterans Health Administration and HRSA. HRSA-supported health centers serve over 19 million patients a year (HRSA, 2011) and provide a safety net for society's most vulnerable populations. Although most primary care is delivered through the private sector, both private and government-supported primary care share common features: both are person- rather than disease-focused, provide a point of first contact for whatever people might consider a health or health care problem, are comprehensive, and coordinate care (Starfield and Horder, 2007).

### Public Health

The committee adopted a definition of public health that likewise was borrowed from an earlier IOM report: "fulfilling society's interest in assuring conditions in which people can be healthy" (IOM, 1988, p. 140). To meet this definition, public health has shifted its primary focus from addressing infectious disease to tackling chronic disease. To ensure healthy conditions, public health encompasses a diverse group of public and private stakeholders (including the health care delivery system) working in a variety of ways to contribute to the health of society. Uniquely positioned among these stakeholders is governmental public health. Because health departments are legally tasked with providing essential public health services, they are required to work with all sectors of the community. This allows them to serve as a catalyst for engaging multiple stakeholders to confront community health problems. In addition, their assessment and assurance functions put them in close contact with the community and in touch with the community's health needs. While public health defined broadly in this report goes beyond governmental public health, the committee recognized that health departments play a fundamental role in creating healthy communities and focused on them when possible.

### Integration

While integration can be an imprecise term, integration of primary care and public health was defined for this report as the linkage of programs and activities to promote overall efficiency and effectiveness and achieve gains in population health. The committee conceived of integration in terms of multiple variables—levels, partners, actions, and degree. For this report, the agency and local levels are discussed. Partners for the agency level include HRSA, CDC, and other agencies as necessary; partners for the local level

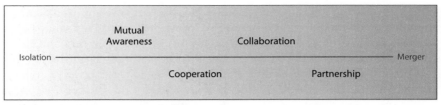

**FIGURE S-1** Degrees of integration.

include a primary care entity, a public health entity (with a preference for health departments), the community, and other stakeholders as necessary. The variable of actions required a shared goal of improved population health; a willingness and ability to contribute to that goal; and, ideally, a commitment to an ongoing process and continual dialogue. Finally, the committee conceived of integration as degrees on a continuum ranging from isolation to merger (Figure S-1) and focused on mutual awareness, cooperation, collaboration, and partnership, with a preference for activities moving toward greater integration.

## CONTEXT FOR INTEGRATION OF PRIMARY CARE AND PUBLIC HEALTH

The opportunity currently exists to shift the health system in significant ways. A number of relatively new developments have converged to create this opportunity. The dramatic rise in health care costs has led many stakeholders to explore innovative ways of reducing costs and improving health. As health research continues to clarify the importance of social and environmental determinants of health and the impact of primary prevention, there is growing recognition that the current model of investment in the nation's health system is unacceptable. At the same time, an unprecedented wealth of health data is providing new opportunities to understand and address community-level health concerns. And most important, the passage of the ACA presents an overarching opportunity to change the way health is approached in the United States.

This pivotal time makes it possible to achieve sustainable improvements in population health, a key goal for health system reform. Pursuit of this goal will require a balance of investment and clarity of roles across activities that address the broad determinants of health, population-level behaviors, and individual health care—activities in which primary care and public health have prominent roles.

Primary care and public health presently operate largely independently, but have complementary functions and the common goal of ensuring a healthier population. By working together, primary care and public health can each achieve their own goals and simultaneously have a greater impact on the health of populations than either of them would have working independently. Each has knowledge, resources, and skills that can be used to assist the other in carrying out its roles. They should be viewed as "two interacting and mutually supportive components" of a health system designed to improve the health of populations (Welton et al., 1997, p. 262).

Among agencies within the Department of Health and Human Services (HHS), HRSA and CDC have especially important roles to play in improving population health. Both have articulated a vision of how their work can impact the broader determinants of health (Frieden, 2010; HRSA, 2010), and both see themselves as having a public health mission. HRSA plays a strategic role in helping to ensure access to personal health services for uninsured and vulnerable populations through its support for the provision of primary care and preventive services at health centers, Ryan White clinics, and rural health clinics, as well as training programs for the primary care and public health workforces and maternal and child health programs. And with its focus on health promotion, disease prevention, and preparedness, CDC is recognized as a global leader in public health. The agency works with local and state health departments on a number of efforts, including implementing disease surveillance systems, preventing and controlling infectious and chronic diseases, reducing injuries, eliminating workplace hazards, and addressing environmental health threats. It is significant that these agencies have come forward to pursue integration.

## PRINCIPLES FOR INTEGRATION

To gain an understanding of current and recent efforts to integrate primary care and public health, the committee reviewed past integration efforts to identify some of the ways in which primary care and public health can interact, as well as the benefits of and barriers to successful collaboration. The committee gathered examples of integration by searching peer-reviewed journal and grey literature databases, querying relevant stakeholders, and drawing on its members' own experiences. A thorough review of these examples revealed some prominent themes and lessons and made it possible to select case studies that reflect the major components of successful integration. The review informed the development of a set of principles that the committee believes are essential for successful integration of primary care and public health:

- a shared goal of **population health improvement;**
- **community engagement** in defining and addressing population health needs;

- **aligned leadership** that
  — bridges disciplines, programs, and jurisdictions to reduce frag-
    mentation and foster continuity,
  — clarifies roles and ensures accountability,
  — develops and supports appropriate incentives, and
  — has the capacity to manage change;
- **sustainability,** key to which is the establishment of a shared infrastructure and building for enduring value and impact; and
- the sharing and collaborative use of **data and analysis.**

While the committee believes that all of these principles are ultimately necessary for integration, it also believes that integration can start with any
of these principles and that starting is more important than waiting until
all are in place.

## EXAMPLES OF INTEGRATION

From the literature review, the committee identified a number of examples of successful integration efforts. These examples appear in a diverse
array of communities and help demonstrate the breadth of possibilities for
primary care and public health interactions. Drawing on these experiences,
the committee derived some lessons about the composition and focus of
recent efforts to integrate primary care and public health:

- In many of the examples, integration was driven by a specific
  health issue that was identified as a community area of concern,
  such as chronic disease, prevention, or the health needs of a specific
  population.
- Participants in integration initiatives varied widely, including an
  array of primary care and public health entities and other contributors, such as community organizations, academic institutions,
  businesses, and hospitals.
- Key opportunities for integration included the sharing and use of
  data and the development of a workforce capable of functioning
  in an integrated environment.

Through its review of the literature, the committee sought examples
to use as case studies that would demonstrate well-developed relationships
between public health and primary care. With these examples, the committee wished to highlight ongoing linkages between primary care and public
health entities that extend beyond a single project, demonstrate a commitment to an ongoing relationship between the two disciplines, and reflect the

above principles for integration. The committee selected three communities to showcase:

- Durham, North Carolina;
- San Francisco, California; and
- New York, New York.

## AREAS IN WHICH HRSA AND CDC CAN STRENGTHEN INTEGRATION

To explore the potential for interagency collaboration to foster the integration of primary care and public health, the committee examined how HRSA-supported primary care systems and public health departments could integrate efforts in three specific areas: maternal and child health (specifically the Maternal, Infant, and Early Childhood Home Visiting Program), cardiovascular disease prevention, and colorectal cancer screening. These areas were selected because they lend themselves to a life-course perspective, include elements of mental and behavioral health, and touch on issues relevant to health disparities. They also represent a mix of programs led by HRSA and CDC.

In its review of these three areas (discussed in Chapter 3), the committee was struck by two things. First is the vastly different organizational structures of HRSA and CDC, which create logistical barriers to the formation of partnerships. These structural differences mean there often is no natural link between the agencies. This situation is not necessarily negative. In fact, like puzzle pieces that fit into place, these structural differences can actually assist in promoting better coordination. In the short run, however, the differences can mean that staff from one agency do not always have a natural counterpart in the other. Second, despite these barriers, there is a genuine willingness among the two agencies to work together.

The committee's examination of the above three areas revealed some key ways in which integration can be encouraged. They include the value of using community health workers, the opportunities provided by data sharing, and the possibility of a third party to foster integration. The committee encourages HRSA and CDC to explore these possibilities in the three areas examined by the committee, as well as others.

## POLICY AND FUNDING OPPORTUNITIES

Federal policy and funding are the greatest levers available to HRSA and CDC for encouraging the integration of primary care and public health on the ground. As the most ambitious health policy in a generation, the ACA provides an unusual opportunity to work toward that goal. While the

ACA does not explicitly address the integration of primary care and public health, it provides a menu of initiatives that agencies and communities can exploit to make gains in improving population health.

The ACA authorizes HRSA and CDC to launch a number of new programs that on their own merit promise to be noteworthy, but if coordinated and managed collaboratively from their inception could generate significant momentum in population health at the national, state, and local levels. Particularly promising provisions of the act (highlighted in Chapter 4) fall into four categories—community investments and benefits, coverage reforms, health care transformation, and reshaping the workforce. These provisions are summarized in Table S-1.

**TABLE S-1** Selected Provisions of the Patient Protection and Affordable Care Act That Offer Opportunities for HRSA and CDC

| Affordable Care Act Provision | HRSA and CDC Opportunities |
| --- | --- |
| Community Transformation Grants (ACA §§ 4002 and 4201) The provision authorizes and funds community transformation grants to improve community health activities and outcomes. | • Given that Community Transformation Grants can be viewed as the public health counterpart to the Centers for Medicare & Medicaid Services (CMS) Innovation Center (CMMI) pilots, HRSA and CDC should be aware of the communities where both of these programs are involved. <br> • As community resources for wellness improve through the Transformation Grant system, it may be possible to encourage state and local health department recipients to develop linkages with primary care providers as a central focus of their program planning. <br> • CDC could also begin to link those resources to CMMI pilots, which must be able to link their patients and physician practices with community resources. |
| Community Health Needs Assessments (ACA § 9007) The provision amends the Internal Revenue Code by adding new section 501(r), "additional requirements for certain hospitals." The new requirements apply to all facilities licensed as hospitals and organizations recognized by the Treasury secretary as hospitals and spell out new obligations for all hospitals seeking federal tax exempt status. | • HRSA and CDC could engage with community hospitals and national hospital associations to develop approaches to hospital community benefit planning, as well as promote approaching jointly the selection of interventions and implementation strategies to address identified problems—for example, the extension of primary care services into nontraditional settings; the formation of collaboratives among community primary care providers and local public health and other agencies; and community health promotion activities involving diet, exercise, and injury risk reduction, as well as other population-level interventions. |

**TABLE S-1** Continued

| Affordable Care Act Provision | HRSA and CDC Opportunities |
|---|---|
| Medicaid Preventive Services (ACA §§ 4106 and 2001) (ACA § 4108) The provision gives states the option to improve coverage of clinical preventive services for traditional eligibility groups, as well as Medicaid benchmark coverage for newly eligible persons, redefined to parallel the act's definition of essential health benefits, which includes coverage for preventive services. It also provides Medicaid incentives for prevention of chronic diseases. | • Primary care providers and public health departments could become participating Medicaid providers and collaborate in designing programs to furnish preventive services to adult and child populations. <br> • HRSA and CDC could collaborate with CMS on the development of joint guidance regarding coverage of preventive services. Such guidance might explain both the required and optional preventive service provisions of the law, as well as federal financing incentives for coverage of those services. Such guidance also might describe best practices in making preventive services more accessible to Medicaid beneficiaries through the use of expanded managed care provider networks and out-of-network coverage in nontraditional locations such as schools, public housing, and workplace sites; qualification criteria for participating providers; recruitment of providers; measurement of quality performance; and assessment of impact on population health. <br> • HRSA and CDC have a crucial role to play in the implementation of state demonstrations, particularly in outreach to community providers to enlist them as active participants in such demonstrations, training and technical support to state Medicaid agencies, outreach to public health departments and health centers in demonstration states, and collaboration with CMS on the development of outcome standards and scalability criteria. |
| Community Health Centers (ACA § 5601) The provision expands funding for health centers. | • An imperative for HRSA is to preserve and strengthen the role of health centers as core safety net providers of clinical care and prevention in the communities they serve. Incentives could be built into funding for these centers to promote activities and linkages with local public health departments and encourage community engagement and partnerships for community-based prevention. <br> • Outreach campaigns to promote clinical preventive services in underserved communities, as well as initiatives aimed at improving the quality of primary care for populations with serious and chronic health conditions, could focus on how to improve the performance of health centers. |

*continued*

**TABLE S-1** Continued

| Affordable Care Act Provision | HRSA and CDC Opportunities |
|---|---|
| National Prevention, Health Promotion and Public Health Council and the National Prevention Strategy (ACA § 4001) The provision creates the National Prevention, Health Promotion and Public Health Council to create a collaborative national strategy to address health in the nation. | • HRSA and CDC could use the Council as a mechanism for working with other agencies around the integration of primary care and public health. |
| CMS Innovation Center (CMMI) (ACA § 3021) The provision establishes CMMI to develop, conduct, and evaluate pilots for improving quality, efficiency, and patient health outcomes in both the Medicare and Medicaid programs, with an emphasis on dual enrollees. | • HRSA and CDC could engage with CMMI in the implementation of its community health innovation program to develop models that would leverage clinical care to achieve a broader impact on population health. <br> • In the CMMI provisions of the ACA and elsewhere in the act, a major thrust of health care reform is attention to dually eligible Medicare/Medicaid beneficiaries. HRSA and CDC could develop an initiative aimed at improving the health and health care of this population. |
| Accountable Care Organizations (ACOs) (ACA § 3022) The provision authorizes the secretary of the Department of Health and Human Services (HHS) to enter into agreements with ACOs on a shared savings basis to improve the quality of patient care and health outcomes and increase efficiency. | • HRSA could encourage health centers to form ACOs and link with public health departments in this endeavor. <br> • HRSA and CDC could develop models of collaboration between public health departments and ACOs that include safety net providers. Such models might emphasize the role of public health in needs assessment, performance measurement and improvement, health promotion, and patient engagement, all of which are central elements of ACOs. |

## TABLE S-1 Continued

| Affordable Care Act Provision | HRSA and CDC Opportunities |
| --- | --- |
| Patient-Centered Medical Homes (ACA § 3502) The provision authorizes state Medicaid programs to establish medical homes for Medicaid beneficiaries with chronic health conditions, and authorizes the secretary of HHS to award grants for the establishment of health teams to support primary care. | • HRSA and CDC could collaborate on further development of the medical home model and its team-based approach to care and encourage the inclusion of local public health departments in that model.<br>• HRSA and CDC could provide technical support to state Medicaid agencies seeking to pursue the medical home model, imparting best practices in the design and development of a medical home that is comprehensive, efficient in care delivery, and patient/family-centered. This support also could be expanded to include the development of performance measurement tools for measuring progress in these areas.<br>• HRSA and CDC could develop a sustainable model for the medical home in Medicare and Medicaid that encourages inclusion of local public health departments, supports multiple population types, and can be translated for private health insurance as well. |
| Primary Care Extension Program (ACA § 5405) The provision authorizes the Agency for Healthcare Research and Quality (AHRQ) to award competitive grants to states for the establishment of Primary Care Extension Programs to improve the delivery of primary care and community health. | • HRSA and CDC could work with AHRQ to ensure that Primary Care Extension Programs include a public health orientation and integrate community health issues into practice- and clinic-based primary care improvement activities.<br>• HRSA and CDC, working jointly with AHRQ, could seek collaboration with CMMI to fund Primary Care Extension Program models for which there is evidence for improving personal and population health. |
| National Health Service Corps (ACA § 5207) The provision expands funding for the National Health Service Corps. | • HRSA and CDC could collaborate in prioritizing the recruitment and placement of National Health Service Corps resources and developing linkages with existing Epidemic Intelligence Service (EIS) officers placed in state and local health departments. |

*continued*

**TABLE S-1** Continued

| Affordable Care Act Provision | HRSA and CDC Opportunities |
|---|---|
| Teaching Health Centers (ACA § 5508) The provision authorizes and funds the establishment of and ongoing operational support for teaching health centers, which must be community-based. | • HRSA could work with teaching health centers to adopt the patient-centered medical home curriculum and ensure that any curriculum used to train residents includes strong community and public health components—ideally with residents working on projects that concretely promote primary care-public health integration. • HRSA and CDC could work with the centers on training programs that would be aimed at producing competency to work in community health teams, given the emphasis placed on teams under the ACA. |

NOTE: ACA = Patient Protection and Affordable Care Act.

Despite these opportunities, the current funding system for primary care and public health is not well positioned to promote integration. For example, competing funding streams have the effect of creating silos at the local level rather than encouraging cooperation across entities. Similarly, most funding streams from HRSA and CDC are inflexible, limiting what local entities can do with the funds and how they could be used for integration. Finally, it should be noted that the funds available to HRSA and CDC for supporting and integrating primary care and public health are quite small relative to the funds available to the Centers for Medicare & Medicaid Services (CMS). By joining forces, the three agencies could create much greater momentum toward integration.

## RECOMMENDATIONS

In the committee's view, the principles for integration outlined above serve as a framework for action. The committee developed five recommendations—aimed at the agency and department levels—whose implementation would assist the leadership of CDC, HRSA, and HHS in creating an environment that would support the broader application of these principles.

### Agency Level

**Recommendation 1. To link staff, funds, and data at the regional, state, and local levels, HRSA and CDC should:**

- **identify opportunities to coordinate funding streams in selected programs and convene joint staff groups to develop grants, requests for proposals, and metrics for evaluation;**

- create opportunities for staff to build relationships with each other and local stakeholders by taking full advantage of opportunities to work through the 10 regional HHS offices, state primary care offices and association organizations, state and local health departments, and other mechanisms;
- join efforts to undertake an inventory of existing health and health care databases and identify new data sets, creating from these a consolidated platform for sharing and displaying local population health data that could be used by communities; and
- recognize the need for and commit to developing a trained workforce that can create information systems and make them efficient for the end user.

Recommendation 2. To create common research and learning networks to foster and support the integration of primary care and public health to improve population health, HRSA and CDC should:

- support the evaluation of existing and the development of new local and regional models of primary care and public health integration, including by working with the CMS Innovation Center (CMMI) on joint evaluations of integration involving Medicare and Medicaid beneficiaries;
- work with the Agency for Healthcare and Research Quality's (AHRQ's) Action Networks on the diffusion of best practices related to the integration of primary care and public health; and
- convene stakeholders at the national and regional levels to share best practices in the integration of primary care and public health.

Recommendation 3. To develop the workforce needed to support the integration of primary care and public health:

- HRSA and CDC should work with CMS to identify regulatory options for graduate medical education funding that give priority to provider training in primary care and public health settings and specifically support programs that integrate primary care practice with public health.
- HRSA and CDC should explore whether the training component of the Epidemic Intelligence Service (EIS) and the strategic placement of assignees in state and local health departments offer additional opportunities to contribute to the integration of primary care and public health by assisting community health programs supported by HRSA in the use of data for improving community health. Any opportunities identified should be utilized.

- HRSA should create specific Title VII and VIII criteria or preferences related to curriculum development and clinical experiences that favor the integration of primary care and public health.
- HRSA and CDC should create all possible linkages among HRSA's primary care training programs (Title VII and VIII), its public health and preventive medicine training programs, and CDC's public health workforce programs (EIS).
- HRSA and CDC should work together to develop training grants and teaching tools that can prepare the next generation of health professionals for more integrated clinical and public health functions in practice. These tools, which should include a focus on cultural outreach, health education, and nutrition, can be used in the training programs supported by HRSA and CDC, as well as distributed more broadly.

### Department Level

Recommendation 4. To improve the integration of primary care and public health through existing HHS programs, as well as newly legislated initiatives, the secretary of HHS should direct:

- CMMI to use its focus on improving community health to support pilots that better integrate primary care and public health and programs in other sectors affecting the broader determinants of health;
- the National Institutes of Health to use the Clinical and Translational Science Awards to encourage the development and diffusion of research advances to applications in the community through primary care and public health;
- the National Committee on Vital and Health Statistics to advise the secretary on integrating policy and incentives for the capture of data that would promote the integration of clinical and public health information;
- the Office of the National Coordinator to consider the development of population measures that would support the integration of community-level clinical and public health data; and
- AHRQ to encourage its Primary Care Extension Program to create linkages between primary care providers and their local health departments.

Recommendation 5. The secretary of HHS should work with all agencies within the department as a first step in the development of a national strategy and investment plan for the creation of a primary care and public health infrastructure strong enough and appropriately integrated to enable the agencies to play their appropriate roles in furthering the nation's population health goals.

## REFERENCES

Frieden, T. R. 2010. A framework for public health action: The health impact pyramid. *American Journal of Public Health* 100(4):590-595.

HRSA (Health Resources and Services Administration). 2010. *Public Health Steering Committee recommendations: Reinvigorating HRSA's public health agenda.* Washington, DC: HRSA.

HRSA. 2011. *Uniform Data System 2010 national data.* Washington, DC: Bureau of Primary Care, HRSA, U.S. Department of Health and Human Services.

IOM (Institute of Medicine). 1988. *The future of public health.* Washington, DC: National Academy Press.

IOM. 1996. *Primary care: America's health in a new era.* Washington, DC: National Academy Press.

Kindig, D., and G. Stoddart. 2003. What is population health? *American Journal of Public Health* 93(3):380-383.

Starfield, B., and J. Horder. 2007. Interpersonal continuity: Old and new perspectives. *British Journal of General Practice* 57(540):527-529.

Welton, W. E., T. A. Kantner, and S. M. Katz. 1997. Developing tomorrow's integrated community health systems: A leadership challenge for public health and primary care. *Milbank Quarterly* 75(9184684):261-288.

# 1

# Introduction

Health is influenced by an array of factors, including social, genetic, environmental, and other factors that cut across a number of different sectors. Improving the health of populations therefore will require a collaborative, intersectoral effort that involves public and private organizations and individuals. At the same time, both health problems and community needs, resources, and circumstances vary among localities, so no single approach to combating health problems can be applied.

Primary care and public health are uniquely positioned to play critical roles in tackling the complex health problems that exist both nationally and locally. They share a similar goal of health improvement and can build on this shared platform to catalyze intersectoral partnerships designed to bring about sustained improvements in population health. In addition, they have strong ties at the community level and can leverage their positions to link community organizations and resources. Thus, the integration of primary care and public health holds great promise as a way to improve the health of society. The purpose of this report is to explore how this promise can be realized.

## CURRENT OPPORTUNITIES

It is well documented that the nation's health system is expensive and does not translate into excellent outcomes for all (AHRQ, 2011; United Health Foundation, 2011). The opportunity currently exists to shift the system in significant ways to improve on this situation. Investments in the current model of health care are not focused in the most effective way.

While these patterns of investment have produced what is arguably the best biomedical research and specialty care system in the world, the nation has failed to balance its investments in primary care, public health, prevention, and the broader determinants of health, a problem clearly demonstrated by its low rankings in overall health status. McGinnis and Foege (1993) estimated that nearly half of all U.S. deaths that occurred in 1990 were attributable to behavioral and environmental factors. It has repeatedly been shown that such factors have a substantial influence on health outcomes, yet the current health system devotes most of its resources to treating disease and much less to the underlying causes of illness (CDC, 1992; Miller et al., 2012). Financial incentives and a medical culture focused overly on acute care and heroic cures encourage giving most attention to individuals who are already sick rather than promoting an effective balance of treatment and personal and community-based prevention. As a result, the current health system is inadequately equipped to provide critical health promotion and preventive services.

A number of relatively new developments have converged to create opportunities for improving the nation's health. First, there is growing recognition that the status quo is unacceptable. The unsustainable rise in health care costs has created an urgent need for innovative ways to deliver health care more efficiently. This imperative has been evident not only in the activities of government health organizations but also in the private sector. As purchasers of health care, many employers have been exploring ways to reduce the growth in these costs. A recent survey by Towers Watson and National Business Group on Health (2010) found that many employers are incentivizing a number of healthy lifestyle activities for their employees, including weight management, smoking cessation, and screenings. The concern about health care expenditures has opened the door for innovative approaches to improving health and health care.

Adding momentum to the recognition that the status quo is unacceptable, health research continues to clarify the importance of social and environmental determinants of health (Marmot and Wilkinson, 2006; McMichael, 1999) and the limitations of the acute care medical system in addressing prevention and care needs in chronic illness. At the same time, the science with respect to primary prevention has grown and developed (The New York Academy of Medicine, 2009). As a result of these factors, a shift in the way health is approached in the United States is taking place.

Another development is the increased availability of health-related data. Advances in data collection techniques and health informatics have presented an opportunity to facilitate the utilization and sharing of data among health professionals. Recent endeavors have begun to capitalize on these opportunities. For instance, the Health Information Technology for Economic and Clinical Health (HITECH) Act encourages the collection and use of patient-level data through electronic health records.[1] In addition to improvements in how data are collected and used, more data sets are becoming available for widespread use. And the Health Data Initiative, led by the Department of Health and Human Services (HHS), has made a wide array of health-related data available to the public (HHS, 2011b). These newly available data are providing communities, health care providers, and researchers with an unprecedented opportunity to access and analyze information that can aid in understanding and addressing community-level health concerns. The new opportunities presented by these data give primary care and public health a solid foundation upon which they can initiate integration.

Finally, and most important, the recent national focus on health care reform and the adoption of the Patient Protection and Affordable Care Act (ACA) present an overarching opportunity to change the way health care is organized and delivered. The ACA is discussed in more detail later in the report.

The convergence of these opportunities makes this a pivotal time to achieve sustainable improvements in population health. When discussing the term "population health," the committee chose to adopt Kindig and Stoddart's definition (2003, p. 381): "the health outcomes of a group of individuals, including the distribution of such outcomes within the group." In this report, population health is viewed as an ultimate goal toward which the strategies and reforms discussed in subsequent chapters would move the health system.

## THE PATH TO IMPROVING POPULATION HEALTH

Improving population health will require activities in three domains: (1) efforts to address social and environmental conditions that are the primary determinants of health, (2) health care services directed to individuals, and (3) public health activities operating at the population level to address health behaviors and exposures. There is abundant evidence for the benefit and value of activities in each of these domains for achieving the aim of better and more equitable population health (Andrulis, 1998; Commission on Social Determinants of Health, 2008; WHO, 2003).

A clear challenge for achieving improved population health is generating an appropriate balance in investment across and within these three domains, clarifying the appropriate roles and tasks for stakeholders in each domain, and improving the integration of activities at the interfaces among the domains. It is in this context that primary care and public health have

---

[1] *American Recovery and Reinvestment Act of 2009 (ARRA)*, HR1, Section 13001, 111th Cong. (February 17, 2009).

critical roles. Their integration can not only improve the efficiency and effectiveness of each of their functions but also lead to collaboration with other entities that will assist in the improvement of population health. Integration of primary care and public health can serve as a catalyst for cooperation across the entire health system, connecting key stakeholders in communities nationwide.

## KEY TERMS

To discuss the integration of primary care and public health, it is necessary to understand what these terms mean broadly and how they are used in this report.

### Primary Care

In 1996, the IOM Committee on the Future of Primary Care defined primary care as "the provision of integrated, accessible health care services by clinicians who are accountable for addressing a large majority of personal health care needs, developing a sustained partnership with patients, and practicing in the context of family and community" (IOM, 1996, p. 1). The committee emphasized that "primary" means care that is first and fundamental, and declared that primary care is not a specialty or a discipline but an essential function in health care systems. The inclusion of the words "integrated," "sustained partnership," and "context of family and community" reflects a prominent population perspective, as well as a responsibility to connect with other actors in the health system.

Also embedded in the 1996 report is the inextricable link between mental health and primary care. A paper commissioned for that report, and included as an appendix, asserts that "a sensible vision of primary health care must have mental health care woven into its fabric" (IOM, 1996, p. 285). Primary care providers address a broad range of health issues to which mental health concerns are integral. Mental, behavioral, and physical health are so closely entwined that they must be considered in conjunction with one another. While the nature and role of primary care have been debated and studied at length, it is generally recognized that primary care has the four key features listed in Box 1-1.

The importance of primary care is well known and researched. In their review of the literature, Starfield and colleagues (2005) found that areas with the highest numbers of primary care providers have the best health outcomes; people who consistently receive care from a primary care provider have better health outcomes than those who do not; and the characteristics themselves of primary care are associated with good health. Additionally, primary care was found to be associated with a reduction of

---

**BOX 1-1**
**Four Key Features of Primary Care**

- **It is person- rather than disease-focused.** This focus entails sustained relationships between patients and providers in primary care practices over time, often referred to as continuity.
- **It provides a point of first contact for whatever people might consider a health or health care problem.** In properly organized health care systems, primary care ensures access to needed services.
- **It is comprehensive.** By definition, it can encompass any problem. Many problems in primary care are ambiguous and defy precise diagnosis. Nonetheless, primary care meets a large majority of patient needs without referral.
- **It coordinates care.** Primary care adopts mechanisms that facilitate the transfer of information about health needs and health care over time. Highly personalized solutions to patients' problems can be implemented when sustained relationships permit deeper knowledge and understanding of individuals' habits, preferences, and goals.

SOURCE: Starfield and Horder, 2007.

---

health disparities both in the United States and among international populations (Starfield et al., 2005).

Primary care is the foundation of the U.S. health system. In the United States, more individuals receive care in primary care settings than in any other setting of formal health care. On average, primary care settings see 11 percent of the entire population each month, compared with 1.3 percent for emergency departments and 0.07 percent for academic medical center hospitals (Green et al., 2001). Of interest, these proportions have not changed substantially since the 1950s and 1960s despite the stunning progress of medical knowledge, new technology, and expansion of health services (White et al., 1961).

The primary care system in the United States comprises both private providers and those supported by government agencies, such as the Veterans Health Administration and the Health Resources and Services Administration (HRSA). HRSA-supported health centers serve nearly 20 million patients a year (HRSA, 2011) and provide a safety net for society's most vulnerable populations. Although most primary care is delivered through the private sector, both private and government-supported primary care share common features. For example, in its policy paper on primary care, the National Business Group on Health, which represents more than 300 large employers providing health care coverage for 55 million people, asserts that primary care should be the key to efficiency, effectiveness, and quality improvement in the nation's health system (National Business Group on Health, 2010). Both sectors also share the same challenges.

As a whole, primary care currently is facing a workforce shortage. The primary care workforce remains a relatively small proportion of the overall workforce compared with other health fields (Bodenheimer et al., 2009; Canadian Labour and Business Centre, 2003; European Observatory on Health Systems and Policies, 2006). During the last decade, the proportion of primary care providers fell from nearly a third to now less than a fourth of the output of the graduate medical education system (COGME, 2010; Phillips et al., 2011; Salsberg et al., 2008). This decline goes beyond physicians to include nurse practitioners and physician assistants as well (HRSA, 2010; Jones, 2007). Primary care also faces a chronic problem of relative shortage due to workforce maldistribution (Zhang et al., 2008). Regional shortages have seen little improvement despite federal and state loan repayment programs and the rapid growth of safety net clinics over the last decade (GAO, 2003).

In addition to workforce shortages, the increase in chronic diseases has posed challenges for primary care and served to motivate its transformation. Chronic diseases are linked to a number of unhealthy behaviors, such as lack of physical activity, poor nutrition, and tobacco use, but primary care often has struggled to address these behaviors adequately. In recognition of the difficulties associated with treating chronic diseases, the Chronic Care Model (Wagner et al., 2001) was implemented. This initiative emphasized a systematic and more efficient means of improving chronic care management for individual patients (Coleman et al., 2009). In its fullest expression, the Chronic Care Model contained six critical elements—community resources and policies, health care organization, self-management support, delivery system design, decision support, and clinical information systems—and effectively bridged patient care across the practice setting, the delivery system, and the broader community (Bodenheimer et al., 2002)

The success of the Chronic Care Model in revitalizing the management of patients with chronic conditions by relying on an interdisciplinary primary care team with aligned objectives and methodology generated interest in redesigning the entire practice of primary care. This interest in reinventing primary care led in turn to interest in the "medical home," a model first proposed in the 1960s for providing care for children with special needs (Rosenthal, 2008). In the last few years, intensive activity has focused on implementing the "patient-centered medical home," spurred by funding and research supported by the Centers for Medicare & Medicaid Services (CMS), the Commonwealth Fund, HRSA, and a number of other groups. These efforts are aimed at stimulating new models of care delivery, with primary care teams at the core of the delivery structure.

A fully realized patient-centered medical home encompasses the principle that individual patients are members of a broader community, and that activity within the construct of individual clinical encounters includes links that can be leveraged to generate wellness and prevention beyond the individual patient. A systematic approach to population health, called community-oriented primary care (COPC), is employed in other health systems and has previously been studied by the Institute of Medicine (IOM, 1984). This approach to primary care helped launch the community health center movement in the United States and is still used in some communities. COPC, which is discussed in more detail later in the chapter, offers a model of primary care that more fully embraces public health. There is already some evidence that the foundational relationship between patient and primary care provider can generate dividends for the broader community. Several integrated service delivery networks, such as the Geisinger Health System, Group Health Cooperative of Puget Sound, and HealthPartners, are providing early evidence that accountable care for patient panels and populations can reduce mortality, costs, and unnecessary utilization, and in some cases can improve the fiscal health of hospitals as well (Flottemesch et al., 2011; Grumbach and Grundy, 2010; IOM, 2010).

Primary care is well positioned to work with public health on improving the health of local populations. The research networks of major primary care provider groups could assist in this effort. Some of primary care's major concerns include factors that are not present in a clinical setting, such as circumstances at the onset of illness, predisposing factors that increase the risk of death and disease, and precipitating factors that lead people to seek care (White, 2000). One of its strengths is that primary care often holds a position of trust in communities and is able to leverage that position in addressing community concerns. This community relationship is exemplified by health centers and other primary care delivery systems, particularly those that use a community-oriented approach. Thus, primary care is working in areas that largely overlap with public health and is strategically placed at the interface of people in communities and the rest of the health care system.

## Public Health

Public health is a dynamic field that continues to evolve to meet the needs of society. While the concept of modern public health emerged in response to the conditions that resulted from industrialization and the subsequent rise in infectious diseases (Rosen, 1993), the issues confronting public health look very different today. Although the primary focus of public health has shifted from infectious to chronic diseases, which are more prevalent in today's society, its emphasis has remained on improving conditions where people spend their lives outside of health care settings.

While it is generally recognized that a critical component of public health is the services provided under the legal authority of government through health departments, articulating broadly what public health is and does is no easy task.

A number of key reports published over the last few decades have presented a vision for public health. The 1988 IOM report *The Future of Public Health* provides two critical definitions. The first is the mission of public health, defined as "fulfilling society's interest in assuring conditions in which people can be healthy" (IOM, 1988, p. 140). The second is the substance of public health, defined as "organized community efforts aimed at the prevention of disease and promotion of health. It links many disciplines and rests upon the scientific core of epidemiology" (IOM, 1988, p. 41). Although the report emphasizes the importance of government health agencies and argues that strengthening the role of health departments would be crucial in moving public health forward in the future, its overall conception of public health is much broader, involving the private sector, community organizations, public–private partnerships, and others.

In 2002, the IOM released *The Future of the Public's Health in the 21st Century*, which reinforces the idea that public health's broad mission of ensuring healthy communities requires interactions among a number of health-influencing actors, such as communities, businesses, the media, governmental public health, and the health care delivery system (IOM, 2002). The report notes that health departments are not alone in carrying out the essential public health services listed in Box 1-2. Figure 1-1 depicts

---

**BOX 1-2**
**Essential Public Health Services**

- Monitor health status to identify community health problems.
- Diagnose and investigate health problems and health hazards in the community.
- Inform, educate, and empower people about health issues.
- Mobilize community partnerships to identify and solve health problems.
- Develop policies and plans that support individual and community health efforts.
- Enforce laws and regulations that protect health and ensure safety.
- Link people to needed personal health services, and assure the provision of health care when otherwise unavailable.
- Assure a competent public health and personal health care workforce.
- Evaluate effectiveness, accessibility, and quality of personal and population-based health services.
- Research for new insights and innovative solutions to health problems.

SOURCE: Public Health Functions Steering Committee, 1994.

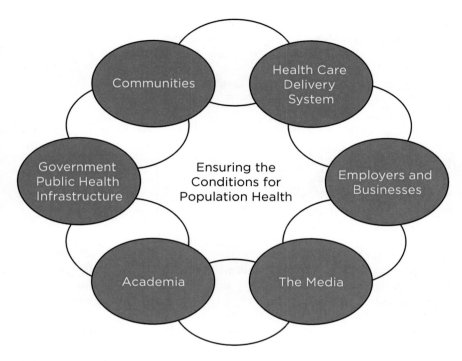

**FIGURE 1-1** The intersectoral public health system.
SOURCE: IOM, 2002.

an interconnected system of sectors that influence a population's health, with government public health being one of several actors (IOM, 2002).

More recently, the IOM published two in a series of reports called *For the Public's Health*, looking at public health in the context of measurement and law (IOM, 2011a,b). A third report, on financing, was published in 2012 (IOM, 2012). These reports provide an opportunity to revisit public health in light of changes in health status in the United States since the IOM's 1988 report was published. For example, obesity tripled among children and doubled among adults between 1980 and 2008 (CDC, 2011). Recognizing the complex nature of health challenges facing society today, the IOM committee responsible for the report on measurement noted that it is the "complex interactions of multiple sectors that contribute to the production and maintenance of the health of Americans" (IOM, 2011b, p. 21). The prevention of disease, which is a pillar of public health's work, requires the engagement of all segments of a community. For instance, combating the rise in obesity requires encouraging individuals to improve their diet and increase physical activity. These efforts require multiple partners, such as schools, employers, urban planners, and policy makers. These various stakeholders may provide one or more of the essential public health services. For example, a community-based organization may implement a health outreach campaign to educate people about health issues, or a public–private partnership may be engaged to mobilize the community to solve a particular health problem.

Traditionally, public health has worked with systems, policy, and the environment to reduce the burden of infectious disease. Improvements in sanitation, food preparation, and water treatment are successful examples of this work. To address more current concerns, public health has turned its attention to fighting chronic disease. Community-based interventions undertaken by public health for the prevention of chronic diseases have proven to be effective (The New York Academy of Medicine, 2009). In addition, some research suggests that making system, policy, and environmental changes may be effective; for example, French and colleagues (2004) found that an intervention aimed at the school environment resulted in students purchasing healthier foods. In general, the field would benefit from additional efforts to evaluate the effectiveness of these interventions in terms of implementation and outcomes.

Public health faces a number of challenges, including insufficient funding to fulfill its mission, a shrinking workforce, and inadequate investments in health information technology (HIT). In its report on public health funding, the Trust for America's Health found that public health funding had been reduced at the federal, state, and local levels (ASTHO, 2011; NACCHO, 2011; Trust for America's Health, 2011). Not surprisingly, a reduction in the public health workforce has also been documented (ASTHO, 2011; NACCHO, 2011; Trust for America's Health, 2011). Another concern for public health is the lack of investment, relative to the health delivery system, in HIT. This disparity is exemplified by the distribution of HIT funding in the American Recovery and Reinvestment Act of 2009, which designated $17.2 billon of the total $19.2 billion appropriated for HIT for incentives to be paid to physicians and hospitals to promote the use of electronic health records (Steinbrook, 2009). This lack of investment could pose challenges for public health in managing population-level data.

Despite these challenges, public health today continues to meet the changing needs of communities. It encompasses a diverse group of public and private stakeholders (including the health care delivery system) working in a variety of ways to contribute to the health of society. Uniquely positioned among these stakeholders is governmental public health. Because health departments are legally tasked with providing the essential public health services, they are required to work with all sectors of the community.

This allows them to serve as a catalyst for engaging multiple stakeholders to confront community health problems. In addition, their assessment and assurance functions put them in close contact with the community and in touch with its health needs. Public health defined broadly is much more than governmental public health, yet health departments play a fundamental role in creating healthy communities.

### Integration

Integration is an imprecise term that encompasses a wide variety of definitions. Accordingly, the committee decided it would be too limiting and not helpful to use a narrow definition. For this report, integration of primary care and public health is defined as the linkage of programs and activities to promote overall efficiency and effectiveness and achieve gains in population health. Because integration can take many forms, the committee chose to think conceptually about the variables that influence integration, which include the level at which it takes place, the partners involved, the actions entailed, and the degree to which integration occurs.

### Levels

Integration can take place on many different levels. For this report, two major levels—the agency and local community levels—are addressed. The agency level refers to HRSA, the Centers for Disease Control and Prevention (CDC), and other federal agencies. Integration at this level involves largely joint efforts among the leadership of these agencies, as well as the appropriate programmatic staff working together.

At the local level, integration efforts are responsive to local health needs and relate to local resources and partners available and willing to work together. While innovative actions are being taken at the local level, many of which are improving the health of local populations, the committee attempted to distinguish clearly between which of these initiatives involve primary care–public health integration and which are innovative but do not necessarily involve integration. The other variables discussed below were used to make this distinction. It should also be noted that at one extreme, either primary care or public health can adopt approaches typical of the other, thereby integrating these functions within an organization. For example, some public health departments deliver primary care. This report, however, focuses on more formal integration efforts between local primary care and public health organizations.

*Partners*

At the agency level, most primary care–public health linkages in this report refer to HRSA and CDC working directly together, although there are some cases in which it would be beneficial for HRSA and CDC to work jointly with other federal agencies. In some cases, it would also make sense to partner with national provider and public health groups. Thus, the partners for the agency level are HRSA; CDC; and, as available and willing, other federal agencies and national groups.

Partners at the local level include a primary care entity (often as part of a larger organized delivery system), a public health entity, and the community. Often, other stakeholders are involved at the local level as well. For this report, the committee conceived of a primary care entity as any entity whose main purpose is the delivery of primary care, but the report also considers larger organized systems that contain entities with this purpose. These could include a solo practice, a group practice, primary care providers affiliated with a health care system, primary care providers affiliated with a university system, a HRSA-supported health center, or other community health centers. The committee was more selective in its choice of public health partners. While many entities provide public health services (including academic health centers and community-based organizations), health departments are legally responsible for provision of the essential public health services. Given that the committee's statement of task explicitly mentions local health departments, the report emphasizes them over other entities in integration efforts. Finally, community participation, which could be facilitated through advisory boards, surveys, or community assessments undertaken by health departments, is critical to any integration efforts at the local level.

In addition to primary care and public health entities, other groups working at the community level are striving for population health improvements. These may include business groups, community-based organizations, public–private partnerships, academic health centers, faith-based groups, or other community-level entities. These groups can play many roles. For example, they may act as neutral conveners, able to link primary care and public health in a balanced way. They may also provide shared resources, such as community health workers, IT support staff, or case managers— resources that neither primary care nor public health may be able to support, but that could be beneficial in linking the two. Thus for the purposes of this report, linkages created at the community level must consist of a primary care partner, a public health partner (preferably a health department), and the community itself. However, other stakeholders working in the community may and often should be involved as well.

*Actions*

How the above partners integrate will differ depending on which partners are involved, the level at which the integration is occurring, and the local situation. At a minimum, each partner should be committed to a shared goal of improved population health and be willing and able to contribute to achieving that goal. The contribution may range from ideas and planning assistance, to financial or human resources, to goods or a physical space, but ideally will include a shared vision for an ongoing and sustainable relationship and a continual dialogue that goes beyond a single project. The contributions of each partner may not always be equal. And the action need not always be challenging; taking on easy tasks to start is as valid as tackling more complex problems. It is the shared recognition that success is not possible without each of the partners that is key.

*Degree*

As stated above, integration can have different meanings for different people. To some, it has a negative connotation, implying that one entity is subsumed by another, stronger entity. To others, integration has a positive connotation, suggesting a seamless flow between two entities. The committee recognized that integration occurs along a continuum (see Figure 1-2). At one end of this continuum is isolation, with primary care and public health entities working completely separately. At the other end is merger, with one combined entity replacing the formerly separate entities. By using the term "integration," the committee is not advocating for a complete merger, nor does it see the benefit of isolation. Rather, the committee believes there are degrees of integration—ranging from mutual awareness, to cooperation, to collaboration, to partnership—that can be used to achieve better health. With mutual awareness, primary care and public health are informed about each other and each other's activities. Cooperation denotes some sharing of resources, such as space, data, or personnel. Collaboration is more intense and involves joint planning and execution, with both enti-

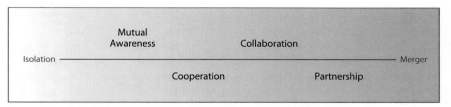

**FIGURE 1-2** Degrees of integration.

ties working together to coordinate at multiple points to carry out a combined effort. Partnership implies integration on a programmatic level, with two entities working so closely together that there is no separation from the end user's perspective; there are, in fact, two parties, but their degree of integration is so great that the effect is nearly seamless. The discussion of integration in this report encompasses all of these degrees. Each community is different, and not all will be able to achieve true partnership. In some communities, achieving mutual awareness will be a significant step forward. However, it is useful to be aware of this continuum and strive for greater integration when possible.

## BENEFITS AND CHALLENGES OF INTEGRATION

Primary care and public health have complementary functions and a common goal of ensuring a healthier population. However, they presently operate largely independently with distinct governance and funding streams, and each approaches this goal differently. Table 1-1, based on a table that highlights the differences between medicine and public health (Fineberg, 2011), provides an overview of these different perspectives.

While their perspectives and approaches may differ, in many ways primary care and public health align neatly. By working together, primary care and public health can each achieve their own goals and simultaneously have a greater impact on the health of populations than either of them would have working independently. For example, public health's ties to community resources can provide support in areas of patient care that are typically difficult for primary care to handle on its own, such as prevention, health promotion, and the management of chronic disease. A primary care practitioner caring for significant numbers of people with asthma can work with local public health agencies to identify geographic areas in the community where poor housing stock or environmental risks can be addressed through combined action with other local stakeholders to remove or reduce asthma risks and ultimately decrease unnecessary use and expense in the health care system. And the incorporation of data from frontline health care providers into public health systems can enable more accurate and timely assessments of health issues, such as infectious disease outbreaks or diseases related to environmental exposures, as well as chronic disease trends in communities that might suggest areas for public health interventions.

These examples illustrate why primary care and public health should and how they could integrate. The evidence base supporting integration is not robust. Few studies have specifically examined integration and gauged its impact on health or process outcomes. In Chapter 2, some examples of integration taking place in local communities around the United States

**TABLE 1-1** Perspectives of Medicine and Public Health

| Medicine | Public Health |
| --- | --- |
| Primary focus on individual | Primary focus on population |
| Personal service ethic, conditioned by awareness of social responsibilities | Public service ethic, tempered by concerns for the individual |
| Emphasis on diagnosis and treatment, care for the whole patient | Emphasis on prevention, health promotion for the whole community |
| Medical paradigm places predominant emphasis on medical care | Public health paradigm employs a spectrum of interventions aimed at the environment, human behavior and lifestyle, and medical care |
| Well-established profession with sharp public image | Multiple professional identities with diffuse public image |
| Biologic sciences central, stimulated by needs of patients; move between laboratory and bedside | Biologic sciences central, stimulated by major threats to health of populations; move between laboratory and field |
| Clinical sciences an essential part of professional training | Clinical sciences peripheral to professional training |
| Rooted mainly in the private sector | Rooted mainly in the public sector |

SOURCE: Based on Fineberg, 2011.

are presented; cases in which improved outcomes have been reported are highlighted.

It has long been asserted that public health and primary care should be viewed as "two interacting and mutually supportive components" of a health system designed to improve the health of populations (Welton et al., 1997, p. 262). There is vast potential for alignment between the two sectors. Each has knowledge, resources, and skills that can be used to assist the other in carrying out its roles. To quote the 1996 IOM report *Primary Care: America's Health in a New Era,* "the population-based functions of public health and the primary care services delivered to individuals are complementary functions, and strengthening the relationship should be the focus of action in both arenas" (pp. 131-132).

## Benefits of Integration

As mentioned above, there have been few formal analyses of the efficacy of primary care and public health integration. However, evidence indicates that some advantages can be realized through integration.

A recent literature review of primary care and public health collaborations conducted in Canada found that these efforts resulted in improved health outcomes, improved workforce outcomes, and benefits at the patient and population levels (Martin-Misener et al., 2009), but that these examples are not widespread. Lasker and the Committee on Medicine and Public Health (1997) conducted a review of more than 400 instances of medicine and public health collaboration and noted a number of benefits that arose from such endeavors. Specifically, the authors found that collaboration benefited clinicians by providing population-based information relevant to their practices, enhancing their capacity to address behaviors and the underlying causes of illness, and generating better quality assurance standards and performance measures. Public health entities received support for their role in carrying out population-based strategies, including the collection of individual-level data for surveillance purposes, the dissemination of health education and key health promotion messages, and cooperation for the assurance of quality medical care for all members of a community.

Beyond the benefits to providers and public health entities, it stands to reason that society gains from integration as well. Integration can improve the efficiencies and harness the capabilities of primary care and public health and their respective workforces to focus on common problems. By joining forces, primary care and public health are better able to meet the nation's goal of improved population health. Unfortunately, however, integration is no easy task.

## Challenges of Integration

Aligning primary care and public health to work together and with other partners in pursuit of the shared goal of improved population health is challenging. A number of trends reinforce the fragmented nature of the current health system, including a history of segregation between primary care and public health, a lack of financial resources and incentives, and an inflexible regulatory system (Baker et al., 2005; IOM, 1988, 2002, 2003, 2011b).

In the early 20th century, despite years spent as related and overlapping areas (Brandt and Gardner, 2000; Duffy, 1979), public health began to establish itself as a profession independent of medicine. This fissure can be traced to a number of factors, most notably the decision to create public health schools separate from medical schools and the rise of the biomedical model.

In 1915, the Welch-Rose Report, authored by William Welch and Wycliffe Rose of the Johns Hopkins School of Medicine, described a research-focused approach to public health education. Based on this report, the Rockefeller Foundation, with which Welch was affiliated, began to focus its philanthropic efforts on public health, and in 1916, the Johns Hopkins School of Hygiene and Public Health was established with financial support from the foundation. By 1947, 10 schools of public health had been established, separating public health education from the more narrowly focused and uniform medical curriculum. As public health professionals and educators argued for more independence from medicine in universities and government, public health became viewed by medical professionals as an economic competitor that was largely encroaching on matters believed to be best resolved through the care and treatment provided by medical professionals to individual patients (Brandt and Gardner, 2000).

In addition to this separation, the biomedical model of disease emerged from a greater understanding of germ theory and bacteriology. This model conceived of disease as something separate from any social causes. As the objective biomedical model gained prominence, a natural consequence was the uncoupling of medical care from public health, which was viewed as being marred by politics and social matters. This view led to a decline in spending on and attention to public health relative to medical care that persists today (Brandt and Gardner, 2000).

After decades of separation, both primary care and public health have hard-won identities, achievements, and cultures that they prize. Revising these identities and adapting to each other's cultures in order to integrate their efforts can be experienced as a loss. Both sectors tend to view themselves as neglected and underappreciated. Both primary care and public health are fragmented within themselves, sometimes struggling to coordinate and align efforts internally, much less with each other. Both have dedicated advocacy groups that stake out territory and defend it against encroachment by alternative interests.

This historical divide is further cemented by a lack of financial investment in both primary care and public health. In this environment, the creation of financial incentives and supporting linkages between primary care and public health is not easy to accomplish or sustain. Payment structures within the delivery system reward disease treatment rather than prevention, pay for volume rather than value, and incentivize specialty care and procedural interventions over primary care. Moreover, primary care and public health both receive a relatively small proportion of the expenditures devoted to health in the United States (as discussed in more detail in Chapter 4). Frequently, they find themselves competing with each other for resources insufficient for either, much less both. Primary care and public health at their best result in nonevents, often at moments distant in time, for individuals and populations, making success somewhat invisible to others. This invisibility often hinders both sectors from attracting funders willing to invest in improvement efforts.

Furthermore, both primary care and public health operate under inflexible regulatory policies and funding restrictions that may preclude or hamper shared action. Neither is accountable to the other, and there is no shared space where primary care and public health come together routinely and automatically to identify problems and opportunities, plan together, coordinate their work, and undertake joint efforts. In terms of informatics and data collection, primary care and public health often lack interoperable information systems both within the delivery system and between the delivery and public health systems. This internal fragmentation and external siloing often means that even when entities are willing to integrate, they lack the infrastructure to do so.

These challenges notwithstanding, the committee believes that the potential benefits of greater integration of primary care and public health are sufficiently promising to merit action now, taking these challenges into account. The call to better integrate primary care and public health is not new. The National Commission on Community Health Services, in a report known as "The Folsom Report" (1966), raised this issue half a century ago by calling for a more comprehensive model of health including both primary care and public health elements; Kerr White's *Healing the Schism* revisited this idea in 1991 (White, 1991). While examples of long-term, successful models of integration are not abundant, there appears to be an interest in communities in bringing primary care and public health together to improve population health (see Box 1-3 and Chapter 2). However, the sustainability and scalability of models of integration have been lacking. The key task now is to focus on the challenge of sustainable implementation of community-based models of primary care and public health integration. Critical elements for this task are providing sustained resources and incentives for these models and supporting the infrastructure necessary to weave together the diverse stakeholders across multiple sectors that must participate in their implementation.

---

**BOX 1-3**
**Interest in Collaboration**

A willingness to collaborate is evident among diverse health disciplines. In 2011, the National Committee on Vital and Health Statistics focused on communities as learning health systems and explored a convenience sample of contemporary examples of local efforts in multiple states to use data to identify and monitor local health needs and problems. Many examples were readily identified and studied in sufficient detail to conclude that, even without formal programs and sufficient infrastructure, these efforts were successful and demonstrated widespread interest in collaboration among community leaders, clinicians, public health departments at various political levels, and academicians to identify local health and health care concerns and new, collaborative ways of responding to them (HHS, 2011a).

## PREVIOUS INTEGRATION EFFORTS

Previous examples of integration of primary care and public health can be found both in the United States and abroad.

### Efforts in the United States

Some prior initiatives have focused on bridging the gap between primary care and public health and the community. For example, efforts have been made in some areas within the United States to adopt COPC models. COPC has been defined as a continual process by which primary health care teams provide care to a defined community on the basis of its assessed health needs through the integration in practice of primary care and public health (IOM, 1984). It is a dynamic, interdisciplinary model for planning, implementing, and evaluating primary care, health promotion, and disease prevention in the community that generally has appealed to practitioners working in underresourced areas with limited access to health care services. The application of COPC in the United States has not been widespread. A recent systematic review found that most articles about COPC did not adhere strictly to the model as originally described (Thomas, 2008). Even with modified models, however, a number of COPC initiatives have been found to generate notable improvements in the delivery of primary care (Merzel and D'Afflitti, 2003; Pickens et al., 2002). COPC models have been implemented internationally as well, with some success (Epstein et al., 2002; Iliffe and Lenihan, 2003).

In 1994 the American Medical Association and the American Public Health Association created the Medicine and Public Health Initiative. This effort began with a task force that met for 2 years and outlined shared agendas in several areas. The task force developed seven major recommendations for collaboration between primary care and public health: (1) engaging the community, (2) changing the education process, (3) creating joint research efforts, (4) devising a shared view of health and illness, (5) working together in health care provision, (6) jointly developing health care assessment measures, and (7) translating initiative ideas into action (Beitsch et al., 2005, p. 150). Other activities of note included a national congress in 1996, the development of a grant program funded by the Robert Wood Johnson Foundation (Cooperative Actions for Health Program, 2001), and a monograph of examples of collaboration (Lasker and the Committee on Medicine and Public Health, 1997).While the initiative was successful in promoting and showcasing efforts at the local level, commitment at the state and national levels ultimately faltered (Beitsch et al., 2005).

Since the Medicine and Public Health Initiative, other, more limited efforts to catalogue and analyze integration initiatives on the ground have been undertaken in the United States. These include a review of public–private partnerships that brought together service delivery networks and coalitions of stakeholders focused on public health and community planning (Bazzoli, 1997), an examination of how organizational characteristics and market conditions contribute to collaborations between either community hospitals or community health centers and public health agencies (Halverson et al., 2000), and the American Medical Association's analysis of effective clinical partnerships between primary care practices and public health agencies (Sloane et al., 2009). While these initiatives point to an enduring interest in integration, they were not part of a sustained effort to promote integration, and none alleviated a steady and persistent relative neglect of both primary care and public health.

## International Efforts

There has been some international recognition of the need to coordinate primary care and public health efforts. In 2003, at a primary care strategic planning meeting held to assess the status of health improvement since the Declaration of Alma Ata (WHO, 1978), the World Health Organization noted that "the emphasis placed on community participation and intersectoral collaboration is especially appropriate now, when so many health issues ... cannot be effectively addressed by health systems working in isolation" (WHO, 2003, p. 16). The ensuing report on that meeting recommended the strengthening of public health functions in primary health care settings. Likewise, a number of countries have made efforts to implement the integration of primary care and public health. A restructuring of the National Health Service in England placed public health professionals in Primary Care Trusts in an attempt to change the way primary care operates (The NHS Confederation, 2004). In 2000, New Zealand announced changes to its health care system that established District Health Boards with responsibility for both primary care and public health (New Zealand Ministry of Health, 2000). Attempts to reform public health currently are under way in Canada, where a 2005 workshop called for the Public Health Agency of Canada to develop stronger collaboration between primary care and public health (Rachlis, 2009). In addition, McMaster University in Ontario initiated a research program to explore the potential for collaboration between primary care and public health and the extent to which such collaborative partnerships currently exist (StrengthenPHC, 2011).

## STUDY PURPOSE AND APPROACH

This study originated in a joint request from HRSA and CDC. With the passage of the ACA, these two agencies, further described in Appendix A, have a unique opportunity to ensure that the provisions they are charged with implementing line up in a way that promotes population health and contributes to an enhanced health system with increased access, improved quality, and reduced costs. These agencies asked the IOM to convene the Committee on Integrating Primary Care and Public Health, whose 17 members include experts in primary health care, state and local public health, service integration, health disparities, HIT, health care finance, health care policy, public health law, workforce education and training, organization management, and child health. Biographical sketches of the committee members are presented in Appendix D.

In clarifying the committee's charge at its first meeting, the sponsors reiterated their interest in receiving practical, actionable recommendations that could assist both agencies in establishing linkages with each other and with other relevant agencies. Box 1-4 presents the committee's statement of task. Funding for the study was provided by HRSA, CDC, and the United Health Foundation.

In conducting the study, the committee held six open and two closed meetings. The open meetings were held in Washington, DC, and Irvine, California, and included 34 presentations. Four of the open meetings were focused on HRSA and CDC and their work in the areas of maternal and child health, cardiovascular disease prevention, and colorectal cancer screening. The agendas for the open meetings can be found in Appendix C. Members of the general public made comments at the open meetings and submitted documents to the committee. The committee also reviewed the published literature, held discussions with HRSA and CDC, and commissioned papers on relevant topics. Finally, a number of consultants assisted the committee; they are listed at the front of the report.

While cardiovascular disease prevention was identified as a required area for the study, the committee's statement of task (Box 1-4) included selecting one or two additional areas. The committee selected maternal and child health (further refined to focus on maternal, infant, and early childhood home visiting) and colorectal cancer screening to complement cardiovascular disease prevention. These three areas flow across the life course and include elements of mental and behavioral health, while also reflecting many of the issues related to health disparities.

## ORGANIZATION OF THE REPORT

This report is organized into five chapters. Chapter 2 summarizes the committee's literature review, presents a set of principles identified by the committee as necessary for the integration of primary care and public health, and highlights examples from around the country of innovative integration programs. Chapter 3 focuses on the Maternal, Infant, and

---

**BOX 1-4**
**Statement of Task**

The Health Resources and Services Administration (HRSA) and the Centers for Disease Control and Prevention (CDC) have requested that the Institute of Medicine convene a committee of experts to examine ways to better integrate public health and primary care to assure healthy communities. The committee's work would ultimately result in an evidence-based, integrated model and other recommendations that would help achieve successful linkages between public health and primary care. As part of its work, the committee will address the following questions:

1. What does the evidence report as the best methods to improve population health and/or reduce health disparities through integrating or connecting public health and primary care?

   A. What are the models and factors that promote and sustain effective integration and connection between public health and primary care?
   B. What are the gaps in evidence?

2. What are the best examples of effective public health and primary care integration and connection that address:

   A. Demonstrated, shared accountability for population health improvement
   B. Optimizing the integration of the public health and primary care workforce
   C. Collaborative governance, financing, and care coordination models including optimizing reimbursement to health departments for clinical and case management (particularly STDs and TB models)
   D. Effective use of health information technology (explore the possible role of health departments as data hubs)
      a. This should include non-patient specific reporting of notifiable conditions and health department notification of primary care providers regarding key community health challenges
      b. This should include patient specific information on
         i. TB, HIV, HBV perinatal immunization—coordination of care and follow-up to improve outcomes
         ii. Primary care systems and public health departments as potential hubs (neutral brokers for the community)
         iii. Sentinel surveillance systems (e.g., autism, birth defects)

---

Early Childhood Home Visiting Program, the Million Hearts initiative, and colorectal cancer screening as examples of how HRSA and CDC can foster and support integration. Chapter 4 describes the policy and funding levers that can promote integration. Finally, Chapter 5 offers conclusions and recommendations. In addition, the report contains four appendixes.

c. This should include recommendations on the barriers and steps to make significant progress on exchanging electronic health record generated information

E. Promotion of integration for the goal of achieving high quality primary care and public health

3. How can HRSA and CDC use Affordable Care Act provisions (e.g., community transformation grants, prevention strategy, quality strategy, community health center expansion, National Health Services Corps, and other workforce programs) to promote integration of public health and primary care?

4. How can HRSA-supported primary care systems (e.g., Federally Qualified Health Centers, Rural Health Clinics, Ryan White Clinics) and state and local public health departments effectively integrate and coordinate to improve cardiovascular disease prevention (which would include obesity, tobacco use, aspirin use, blood pressure and cholesterol management)

A. One to two additional topics based on Committee input that address issues relevant to health disparities or specific populations

a. These should be chosen from among immunization, TB control, STD control, asthma management, falls prevention, behavioral health, SBIRT (screening, brief intervention, and referral to treatment), cancer screening, diabetes mellitus prevention and care, and family planning

5. Within each care area, the committee should address potential actions, needs, or barriers regarding:

A. Science
B. Finance
C. Governance
D. Health information technology
E. Delivery system and practice
F. Policy
G. Workforce education and training

6. What actions should CDC and HRSA take to promote these changes?

The committee should engage relevant stakeholders and perform a comprehensive literature review that includes international experiences, to identify promising practices and gaps in integrating public health and primary care.

Appendix A provides a broad description of HRSA and CDC. Appendix B offers an overview of HRSA-supported primary care systems and health departments. Appendix C contains the committee meeting agendas. Finally, Appendix D contains the committee biosketches.

# REFERENCES

AHRQ (Agency for Healthcare Research and Quality). 2011. *2010 national healthcare quality report.* Rockville, MD: AHRQ.

Andrulis, D. P. 1998. Access to care is the centerpiece in the elimination of socioeconomic disparities in health. *Annals of Internal Medicine* 129(5):412-416.

ASTHO (Association of State and Territorial Health Officials). 2011. *Budget cuts continue to affect the health of Americans: Update May 2011.* Arlington, VA: ASTHO.

Baker, E. L., M. A. Potter, D. L. Jones, S. L. Mercer, J. P. Cioffi, L. W. Green, P. K. Halverson, M. Y. Lichtveld, and D. W. Fleming. 2005. The public health infrastructure and our nation's health. *Annual Review of Public Health* 26(1):303-318.

Bazzoli, G. J. 1997. Public-private collaboration in health and human service delivery: Evidence from community partnerships. *Milbank Quarterly* 75(4):533-561.

Beitsch, L. M., R. G. Brooks, J. H. Glasser, and Y. D. Coble. 2005. The medicine and public health initiative: Ten years later. *American Journal of Preventive Medicine* 29(2):149-153.

Bodenheimer, T., E. H. Wagner, and K. Grumbach. 2002. Improving primary care for patients with chronic illness. *Journal of the American Medical Association* 288(14):1775-1779.

Bodenheimer, T., K. Grumbach, and R. Berenson. 2009. Health care 2009: A lifeline for primary care. *The New England Journal of Medicine* 36(26):2693-2696.

Brandt, A. M., and M. Gardner. 2000. Antagonism and accommodation: Interpreting the relationship between public health and medicine in the United States during the 20th century. *American Journal of Public Health* 90(5):707-715.

Canadian Labour and Business Centre. 2003. *Physician workforce in Canada: Literature review and gap analysis.* Ottawa, ON: A Physician Human Resource Strategy for Canada: Task Force Two.

CDC (Centers for Disease Control and Prevention). 1992. Effectiveness in disease and injury prevention estimated national spending on prevention—United States, 1988. *Morbidity and Mortality Weekly Reports* 41(29):529-531.

CDC. 2011. *Obesity: Halting the epidemic by making health easier.* Atlanta, GA: CDC.

COGME (Council on Graduate Medical Education). 2010. *Council on Graduate Medical Education 20th report: Advancing primary care.* Hyattsville, MD: COGME.

Coleman, K., B. T. Austin, C. Brach, and E. H. Wagner. 2009. Evidence on the chronic care model in the new millennium. *Health Affairs* 28(1):75-85.

Commission on Social Determinants of Health. 2008. *Closing the gap in a generation: Health equity through action on the social determinants of health.* Geneva, Switzerland: WHO.

Cooperative Actions for Health Program. 2001. *Lessons learned in medicine and public health collaboration.* Chicago, IL: American Medical Association and Washington, DC: American Public Health Association.

Duffy, J. 1979. The American medical profession and public health: From support to ambivalence. *Bulletin of the History of Medicine* 53(Spring):1-22.

Epstein, L., J. Gofin, R. Gofin, and Y. Neumark. 2002. The Jerusalem experience: Three decades of service, research, and training in community-oriented primary care. *American Journal of Public Health* 92(11):1717-1721.

European Observatory on Health Systems and Policies. 2006. *The health care workforce in Europe learning from experience.* Trowbridge, Wilts: European Observatory on Health Systems and Policies.

Fineberg, H. V. 2011. Public health and medicine. *American Journal of Preventive Medicine* 41(4):S149-S151.

Flottemesch, T. J., P. Fontaine, S. E. Asche, and L. I. Solberg. 2011. Relationship of clinic medical home scores to health care costs. *The Journal of Ambulatory Care Management* 34(1):78-89.

French, S. A., M. Sory, J. A. Fulkerson, and P. Hannan. 2004. An environmental intervention to promote lower-fat food choices in secondary schools: Outcomes of the tacos study. *American Journal of Public Health* 94(9):1507-1512.

GAO (General Accounting Office). 2003. *Physician workforce: Physician supply increased in metropolitan and nonmetropolitan areas but geographic disparities persisted.* Washington, DC: GAO.

Gostin, L. O., P. D. Jacobson, K. L. Record, and L. E. Hardcastle. 2011. Restoring health to public reform: Integrating medicine and public health to advance the population's wellbeing. *Pennsylvania Law Review* 159:1777-1823.

Green, L. A., G. E. Fryer, B. P. Yawn, D. Lanier, and S. M. Dovey. 2001. The ecology of medical care revisited. *New England Journal of Medicine* 344(26):2021-2025.

Grumbach, K., and P. Grundy. 2010. *Outcomes of implementing patient centered medical home interventions: A review of the evidence from prospective evaluation studies in the United States.* Washington, DC: Patient Centered Primary Care Collaborative.

Halverson, P. K., G. P. Mays, and A. D. Kaluzny. 2000. Working together? Organizational and market determinants of collaboration between public health and medical care providers. *American Journal of Public Health* 90(12):1913-1916.

HHS (Department of Health and Human Services). 2011a. *The community as a learning system for health: Using local data to improve local health.* Hyattsville, MD: HHS.

HHS. 2011b. *Health data initiative.* http://www.hhs.gov/open/initiatives/hdi/index.html (accessed September 22, 2011).

HRSA (Health Resources and Services Administration). 2010. *The registered nurse population: Findings from the 2008 national sample survey of registered nurses.* Hyattsville, MD: HHS.

HRSA. 2011. *Uniform Data System 2010 National Data.* Hyattsville, MD: HHS.

Iliffe, S., and P. Lenihan. 2003. Integrating primary care and public health: Learning from the community oriented primary care model. *International Journal of Health Services* 33(1):85-98.

IOM (Institute of Medicine). 1984. *Community oriented primary care: A practical assessment.* Vol. 1. Washington, DC: National Academy Press.

IOM. 1988. *The future of public health.* Washington, DC: National Academy Press.

IOM. 1996. *Primary care: America's health in a new era.* Washington, DC: National Academy Press.

IOM. 2002. *The future of the public's health in the 21st century.* Washington, DC: The National Academies Press.

IOM. 2003. *Who will keep the public healthy? Educating public health professionals for the 21st century.* Washington, DC: The National Academies Press.

IOM. 2010. *The healthcare imperative: Lowering costs and improving outcomes: Workshop series summary.* Washington, DC: The National Academies Press.

IOM. 2011a. *For the public's health: Revitalizing law and policy to meet new challenges.* Washington, DC: The National Academies Press.

IOM. 2011b. *For the public's health: The role of measurement in action and accountability.* Washington, DC: The National Academies Press.

IOM. 2012. *For the public's health: Investing in a healthier future.* Washington, DC: The National Academies Press.

Jones, P. E. 2007. Physician assistant education in the United States. *Academic Medicine* 82(9):882-887.

Kindig, D., and G. Stoddart. 2003. What is population health? *American Journal of Public Health* 93(3):380-383.

Lasker, R. D., and the Committee on Medicine and Public Health. 1997. *Medicine and public health: The power of collaboration.* New York: The New York Academy of Medicine.

Marmot, M. G., and R. G. Wilkinson. 2006. *Social determinants of health*. New York: Oxford University Press.

Martin-Misener, R., R. Valaitis, and The Strengthening Public Health Care Through Primary Care and Public Health Collaboration Research Team. 2009. *A scoping literature review of collaboration between primary care and public health: A report to the Canadian Health Services Research Foundation*. Hamilton, ON: StrengthenPHC.

McGinnis, J. M., and W. H. Foege. 1993. Actual causes of death in the United States. *Journal of the American Medical Association* 270(18):2207-2212.

McMichael, A. J. 1999. Prisoners of the proximate: Loosening the constraints on epidemiology in an age of change. *American Journal of Epidemiology* 149(10):887-897.

Merzel, C., and J. D'Afflitti. 2003. Reconsidering community-based health promotion: Promise, performance, and potential. *American Journal of Public Health* 93(4):557-574.

Miller, G., C. Roehrig, P. Hughes-Cromwick, and A. Turner. 2012. What is currently spent on prevention as compared to treatment? In *Prevention vs. Treatment: What's the right balance?*, edited by H. S. Faust, and P. T. Menzel. New York: Oxford University Press. Pp. 37-55.

NACCHO (National Association of County and City Health Officials). 2011. *Local health department job losses and program cuts: Findings from the July 2011 survey*. Washington, DC: NACHHO.

National Association of Community Health Centers. 2009. *Primary care access: An essential building block of health reform*. Bethesda, MD: National Association of Community Health Centers.

National Business Group on Health. 2010. *The health care delivery system should focus on primary care*. Washington, DC: National Business Group on Health.

National Commission on Community Health Services. 1966. *Health is a community affair: Report*. Cambridge, MA: Harvard University Press.

The New York Academy of Medicine. 2009. *A compendium of proven community-based prevention programs*. New York: The New York Academy of Medicine.

New Zealand Ministry of Health. 2000. *The New Zealand health strategy*. Wellington, New Zealand: Ministry of Health.

The NHS Confederation. 2004. *Making a difference: How primary care trusts are transforming the NHS*. London: NHS Confederation.

Noncommunicable Diseases and Mental Health Evidence and Information for Policy World Health Organization. 2003. *Primary health care: A framework for future strategic directions*. Geneva, Switzerland: WHO.

Phillips, R. L., S. C. Petterson, and A. W. Bazemore. 2011. Primary care physician workforce and outcomes. *Journal of the American Medical Association* 306(11):1201-1202.

Pickens, S., P. Boumbulian, R. J. Anderson, S. Ross, and S. Phillips. 2002. Community-oriented primary care in action: A Dallas story. *American Journal of Public Health* 92(11): 1728-1732.

Public Health Functions Steering Committee. 1994. *Public health in America: Vision, mission, and essential services*. Washington, DC: Office of Disease Prevention and Health Promotion.

Rachlis, M. 2009. *Public health and primary health care collaboration: A paper prepared for the public health agency of Canada*. http://www.michaelrachlis.com/publications.php.

Rosen, G. 1993. *A history of public health: Expanded edition*. Baltimore, MD: The Johns Hopkins University Press.

Rosenthal, T. C. 2008. The medical home: Growing evidence to support a new approach to primary care. *The Journal of the American Board of Family Medicine* 21(5):427-440.

Salsberg, E., P. H. Rockey, K. L. Rivers, S. E. Brotherton, and G. R. Jackson. 2008. US residency training before and after the 1997 balanced budget act. *Journal of the American Medical Association* 300(10):1174-1180.

Sloane, P. D., J. Bates, M. Gadon, C. Irmiter, and K. Donahue. 2009. *Effective clinical partnerships between primary care medical practices and public health agencies.* Chicago, IL: American Medical Association.

Starfield, B., and J. Horder. 2007. Interpersonal continuity: Old and new perspectives. *British Journal of General Practice* 57(540):527-529.

Starfield, B., L. Shi, and J. Macinko. 2005. Contribution of primary care to health systems and health. *Milbank Quarterly* 83(3):457-502.

Steinbrook, R. 2009. Health care and the American Recovery and Reinvestment Act. *New England Journal of Medicine* 360(11):1057-1060.

StrengthenPHC. 2011. *Strengthening primary health care through primary care and public health collaboration: About the project.* http://strengthenphc.mcmaster.ca/ (accessed January 4, 2012).

Thomas, G. 2008. A systematic review of COPC: Evidence for effectiveness. *Journal of Health Care for the Poor and Underserved* 19(3):963-980.

Towers Watson and National Business Group on Health. 2010. *Raising the Bar on Health Care: Moving Beyond Incremental Change.* New York: Towers Watson.

Trust for America's Health. 2011. *Investing in America's health: A state-by-state look at public health funding and key health facts.* Washington, DC: Trust for America's Health.

United Health Foundation. 2011. *America's health rankings: A call to action for individuals and their communities.* St. Paul, MN: United Health Foundation.

Wagner, E., B. Austin, C. Davis, M. Hindmarsh, J. Schaefer, and A. Bonomi. 2001. Improving chronic illness care: Translating evidence into action. *Health Affairs* 20(6):64-78.

Welton, W. E., T. A. Kantner, and S. M. Katz. 1997. Developing tomorrow's integrated community health systems: A leadership challenge for public health and primary care. *Milbank Quarterly* 75(9184684):261-288.

White, K. L. 1991. *Healing the schism: Epidemiology, medicine, and the public's health; with foreword by Halfdan Mahler, Frontiers of primary care.* New York: Spinger-Verlag.

White, K. L. 2000. Fundamental research at primary care level. *The Lancet* 355(9218):1904-1906.

White, K. L., T. F. Williams, and B. G. Greenberg. 1961. Ecology of medical care. *New England Journal of Medicine* 265(18):885-892.

WHO (World Health Organization). 1978. *Declaration of Alma-Ata: International conference on primary health care, Alma-Ata, USSR, 6-12 September 1978.* Paper presented at the International Conference on Primary Health Care.

WHO. 2003. *Social determinants of health: The solid facts.* Copenhagen, Denmark: WHO.

Zhang, X., R. L. Phillips Jr, A. W. Bazemore, M. S. Dodoo, S. M. Petterson, I. Xierali, and L. A. Green. 2008. Physician distribution and access: Workforce priorities. *American Family Physician* 15(77):1378.

# 2

# Integration: A View from the Ground

Recognizing that there are no broadly accepted or implemented models of primary care and public health integration, the committee sought to identify promising examples that would both demonstrate the potential for integration and guide the development and implementation of future integration models. To this end, the committee reviewed the published and gray literature. This chapter describes this literature review, presents key principles derived from the review, and highlights examples thus identified in communities across the United States that both embody the key principles and respond to the committee's statement of task.

## PREVIOUS REVIEWS OF INTEGRATION

As part of its literature review, the committee looked for previous reviews of primary care and public health integration. This search yielded only two major efforts that addressed this topic directly, undertaken by McMaster University (Martin-Misener et al., 2009) and the American Medical Association (Sloane et al., 2009). However, a study conducted by Lasker and the Committee on Medicine and Public Health (1997) provided valuable insights into the integration of medicine and public health. The committee believes all three of these studies are worth highlighting.

## McMaster University Review of Primary Care
## and Public Health Collaborations

In 2008, McMaster University conducted a literature review to gain an understanding of and derive lessons from examples of primary care and public health collaborations (Martin-Misener et al., 2009). A rigorous search resulted in a collection of 114 articles, published between 1988 and 2008, that described examples of such collaboration occurring across Canada, the United States, the United Kingdom, Australia, New Zealand, and Western Europe. After reviewing these examples, the authors drew a number of conclusions about why primary care and public health entities have engaged in collaboration, the types of activities typically carried out in such collaborations, and the major facilitators of and barriers to collaboration.

The authors note the wide variety of examples they collected. Differences among localities in organizational structure and community health needs have led primary care and public health to connect in different ways. Collaborative efforts have arisen from policy mandates; from a natural alignment of goals; and in response to specific, shared challenges. These collaborations also have engaged in a broad range of activities. Box 2-1 lists the major areas of activity appearing in the McMaster literature review.

The review also found that some collaborations were more successful than others. From the available literature, the authors derived a number of factors that tended to influence the success of collaborative efforts. Table 2-1 identifies some of the facilitators of and barriers to collaboration across different levels of the health care system.

Successful collaborations were found to result in improvements in health service delivery, funding and resource allocation, and population health outcomes. The authors recommend further research and evaluation of methods for collaboration between primary care and public health.

---

**BOX 2-1**
**Areas of Activity in Primary Care and**
**Public Health Collaborations**

- Community activities
- Health services
- Information systems
- Quality assurance and evaluation
- Prevention
- Teamwork and management

- Professional education
- Social marketing and communication
- Steering and advisory functions
- Evidence-based practice
- Health promotion and education
- Needs assessment and planning

SOURCE: Martin-Misener et al., 2009.

**TABLE 2-1** Facilitators of and Barriers to Primary Care and Public Health Collaboration

|  | Facilitators | Barriers |
|---|---|---|
| Systems Level | • Government endorsement of the value of collaboration<br>• Sustained government funding<br>• Resources available through pooling and sharing<br>• Professional education emphasizing a system-wide approach to working collaboratively | • Lack of stable funding for collaborative projects<br>• Lack of adequate funding for evaluation of collaboration innovations<br>• Separate, entrenched bureaucracies for medical services and public health<br>• Lack of an adequate information structure |
| Organizational Level | • Multiprofessional involvement<br>• Joint planning by primary care, public health, and the community<br>• Clear lines of accountability<br>• Use of a standardized, shared system for collecting data and disseminating information | • Lack of a common agenda or vision<br>• A focus on individuals and short-term results<br>• Resource limitations<br>• Lack of capacity to coordinate and manage disparate, diverse, and large teams<br>• Limited understanding of the needs of communities |
| Interactional Level | • Clear roles and responsibilities for all partners<br>• Trust, tolerance, and respect for partners<br>• Effective communication | • Resistance to change<br>• Competing priorities and agendas<br>• Poor rapport between primary care and public health, as well as with the community<br>• Inadequate understanding of specific roles and interdisciplinary teamwork |

SOURCE: Martin-Misener et al., 2009.

## American Medical Association Review of Partnerships Between Primary Care Practices and Public Health Agencies

In 2009, the American Medical Association and the University of North Carolina conducted a review of partnerships between primary care practices and public health agencies (Sloane et al., 2009). Through a review of the published literature and a qualitative study of 48 programs, the authors examined the structure of successful collaborations and the factors that led to partnership formation. They found that most of the partnerships they reviewed addressed one of three issues: increasing access of underserved individuals and populations to primary care, enhancing prevention resources for individuals and communities, and improving the quality of care for people with chronic diseases (Sloane et al., 2009). Partnerships typically were initiated by public health professionals. Primary care physicians who were receptive to partnership generally embraced a community-based approach to medicine. Incentives for primary care practices and public health agencies to interact included grant requirements that encouraged collaboration, a mutual benefit from collaboration or a shared goal, and positive experiences in prior professional relationships. The more successful partnerships often developed a shared mission with a formalized structure and clearly defined roles. They were driven by strong leadership and established ongoing communication between the two sectors.

### Lasker and the Committee on Medicine and Public Health Review of Medicine and Public Health Collaborations

In 1997, Lasker and colleagues conducted a study of collaborations between medicine and public health to support the Medicine and Public Health Initiative (Lasker and Committee on Medicine and Public Health, 1997). Examples of such collaborations were solicited from medicine and public health professionals, government health agencies, and other relevant stakeholders. The authors collected and reviewed more than 400 examples, and assessed their structure and the relationships involved. A wide variety of organizations were found to have a role in these collaborations. Box 2-2 lists some of the types of organizations that were identified.

These organizations were found to interact in different ways and for different purposes. The authors identified six "synergies" describing the most prominent ways in which resources and skills were combined in a medicine and public health collaboration. Table 2-2 presents these synergies, along with examples of how they are carried out.

It is important to note that the synergies were not exclusive of one

---

**BOX 2-2**
**Types of Organizations Involved in Medicine and Public Health Collaborations**

- Medical practices
- Community-based clinics
- Laboratories and pharmacies
- Hospitals
- Managed care organizations
- Foundations

- Academic institutions
- Professional associations
- Voluntary health organizations
- Community groups
- The media

SOURCE: Lasker and Committee on Medicine and Public Health, 1997.

**TABLE 2-2** Synergies of Medicine and Public Health Collaboration

| Synergy | Examples |
|---|---|
| Improving health care by coordinating services for individuals | • Bring new personnel and services to existing practice sites<br>• Establish "one-stop" centers<br>• Coordinate services provided at different sites |
| Improving access to care by establishing frameworks to provide care for the uninsured | • Establish free clinics<br>• Establish referral networks<br>• Enhance clinical staffing at public health facilities<br>• Shift indigent patients to mainstream medical settings |
| Improving the quality and cost-effectiveness of care by applying a population perspective to medical practice | • Use population-based information to enhance clinical decision making<br>• Use population-based strategies to "funnel" patients to medical care<br>• Use population-based analytic tools to enhance practice management |
| Using clinical practice to identify and address community health problems | • Use clinical encounters to build community-wide databases<br>• Use clinical opportunities to identify and address underlying causes of health problems<br>• Collaborate to achieve clinically oriented community health objectives |
| Strengthening health promotion and health protection by mobilizing community campaigns | • Conduct community health assessments<br>• Mount health education campaigns<br>• Advocate health-related laws and regulations<br>• Engage in community-wide campaigns to achieve health promotion objectives |
| Shaping the future direction of the health system by collaborating around policy, training, and research | • Influence health system policy<br>• Engage in cross-sector education and training<br>• Conduct cross-sector research |

SOURCE: Lasker and Committee on Medicine and Public Health, 1997.

another; rather, an example often reflected more than one synergy. In fact, some of the most successful examples were ones in which partners combined their resources to address multiple concerns.

## THE COMMITTEE'S LITERATURE REVIEW

The purpose of the committee's literature review was twofold: to gain an understanding of the prevalence of and methods employed by current and recent integration efforts, and to identify a small set of illustrative programs from which key principles for successful integration could be derived. To meet those aims, the review was limited to articles describing an operational (not a theoretical) program that was active in 2000 or later and involved some level of interaction between primary care and public health with the goal of improving population health. Both domestic and international examples were included.

To identify such programs, the committee conducted a search of peer-reviewed journal articles using the PubMed and Medline databases. Keywords relating to the overarching topic areas of primary care, public health, integration, and population health were linked in various combinations using Boolean operators. To supplement the formal literature search, the committee also conducted a grey literature search using the New York Academy of Medicine's grey literature database and the National Technical Information Service database. Additionally, examples of integration were solicited by querying committee members, stakeholders (including the Health Resources and Services Administration [HRSA] and the Centers for Disease Control and Prevention [CDC]), advocacy and professional organizations, and researchers who had done work in the field). After an initial scan of titles and abstracts for basic relevancy, more than 3,000 articles or case descriptions were identified. Abstracts and summaries of those articles were reviewed for general appropriateness, and any article or case description that potentially included a useful example of primary care and public health integration was identified for further review. This process yielded 632 articles.

Finally, these remaining articles were carefully read and evaluated based on the strength of linkages between primary care and public health, as well as the robustness of population health outcomes. Preference was given to examples that involved interaction between distinct primary care and public health entities, with an emphasis on the inclusion of health departments. This process yielded a final 100 articles or case descriptions that contained examples of integration for further review.

This set of examples was delivered to commissioned authors Philip Sloane and Katrina Donahue, who assessed them based on:

- scope of the population served;
- length of time the program was/has been in operation;
- degree of collaboration between primary care and public health;
- robustness of the evaluation and outcomes; and
- degree of innovation (using the authors' subjective assessments).

The committee supplemented this analysis with additional examples from its members' own expertise to create a final portfolio of examples.

## Limitations

The most striking aspect of the committee's literature review was the relatively limited number of articles that described robust examples of primary care and public health integration supported by outcomes. This lack of strong examples may be attributable in part to limitations of the review itself. First, an article describing an example of primary care and public health integration may not identify itself as such; rather, integration examples often are presented as a potential solution to a specific health problem or organizational challenge. Therefore, a search tailored to identifying instances of terms related to primary care, public health, and integration used in conjunction with one another potentially could miss many relevant examples. At the outset, in recognition of this potential limitation, the initial search cast a broad net, yielding more than 3,000 results; however, relevant articles may have been overlooked. In an effort to fill some of these gaps, stakeholders, including HRSA and CDC, and committee members were asked to submit additional relevant examples.

A second limitation is that the review was restricted to published articles. There may be a number of effective integration examples in practice that have neither been described nor evaluated in the peer-reviewed literature.

A third limitation is that the articles reviewed often provide brief or incomplete descriptions of programs. Many of these articles were written to highlight a program's impact on specific health outcomes or to describe specific program elements, and articles often were tailored to the perspective of the audience for which they were written—for example, clinical and public health audiences. As a result, it was often difficult to assess the degree and breadth of integration in a program or obtain a complete understanding of the program's impact.

Finally, it is possible that there are fewer examples of integration under way than the committee anticipated, so that fewer were uncovered than was expected.

Based on these limitations, the committee believes that the integration of primary care and public health could be facilitated by increased evaluation efforts. A series of thorough evaluations of integration efforts currently under way would assist in building a knowledge base, which in turn would enable a richer understanding of the processes by which integration can occur successfully and of the outcomes associated with integration.

### Breadth of Examples

Even with the limitations outlined above, the literature contained many promising examples of integration. These examples reflect a wide variety of approaches and highlight a number of ways in which primary care and public health can be aligned to address community health concerns.

### *Focus Areas for Integration*

Many of the integration examples uncovered by the literature review converged around a specific health issue that was identified as a community area of concern. At times these issues were identified by formal community assessments, but more commonly they were recognized by leaders of one or more of the partners using supporting data. The focus of nearly all of these examples fell into one of three categories: chronic disease, prevention and health promotion, or the health of specific populations.

**Chronic disease** Chronic diseases often have a large public health impact and can require the application of a diverse array of care and management techniques. A number of communities have discovered that the actions of primary care or public health alone are not sufficient to effectively mitigate the impact of chronic diseases on population health. Instead, they have endorsed collaborative, coordinated efforts focused on prevention, care, and outreach that have had some positive results. For example, in response to a statewide increase in the prevalence of diabetes and associated complications, the Michigan Department of Community Health implemented the Michigan Diabetes Outreach Network. The network consists of six independent, regional networks that carry out the Department of Community Health's mission to "create innovative partnerships to strengthen diabetes prevention, detection, and treatment" (Constance et al., 2002, p. 54). The regional networks partner with and support health professionals, businesses, and community groups to identify and reduce disparities in diabetes care, strengthen community resources, enhance knowledge of the disease among health care professionals, raise community awareness, and facilitate data collection and use. Activities of the regional networks have included public awareness campaigns; the development of systems for use in medical practice to promote adherence to established care guidelines; the implementation of health professional education and certification programs in diabetes care; and the initiation of a data collection and reporting system for use by home care providers, physician offices, and diabetes support groups. The program has demonstrated improved health outcomes for Michigan residents with diabetes, as well as a dramatic expansion of the reach and prevalence of community awareness events and health professional education programs (Constance et al., 2002).

**Prevention and health promotion** Chapter 1 highlights the importance of prevention and health promotion activities for improving population health. The impact of these types of activities depends on the ability to reach as much of the target population as possible in a meaningful way. Both primary care and public health have critical roles in prevention and health promotion and are positioned to carry out these roles with different sets of resources and relationships within the community. Many of the examples from the literature review show that, by linking primary care, public health, and the community, coordinated, cooperative approaches to prevention and health promotion can expand the reach and effectiveness of such endeavors.

In a number of cases, a public health partner would seek the involvement of primary care providers to assist in a key public health campaign. These collaborative efforts sought to utilize the individual relationship between provider and patient to complement population-level interventions. Some examples include public health personnel training primary care providers to deliver evidence-based behavioral interventions and linking primary care providers to public health and community resources such as tobacco quit-lines (Larson et al., 2006; Rothemich et al., 2010).

Another approach for integrating around prevention involves primary care, public health, and community groups combining efforts to ensure the broad delivery of clinical preventive services at diverse venues throughout communities. Sickness Prevention Achieved through Regional Collaboration (SPARC), a nonprofit agency, implemented this type of method in the New England area (Shenson et al., 2008). In response to low rates of adult vaccination and cancer screening rates in the area, SPARC leadership recognized that primary care alone could not bear the responsibility of ensuring the community-wide delivery of preventive services. Instead, SPARC positioned primary care providers as partners in a community-spanning coalition of public health and community resources. The program brought together public health agencies, hospitals, social service organizations, and advocacy groups to form a network of prevention activities. Coordination among these groups and with primary care helped ensure a broader reach for prevention services and avoided duplication of effort. The inclusion of a variety of community partners led to the development and widespread implementation of innovative approaches tailored to community needs. SPARC's initiatives have been associated with regional improvements in rates of vaccination and cancer screening, and the SPARC coalition-based model has been replicated successfully in other communities (Shenson et al., 2008).

**Health of specific populations** Providing for the health of certain populations, such as the uninsured, who can be difficult to reach, or older persons living alone who require care outside of a health care delivery setting can present challenges that are difficult for either primary care or public health to handle alone. The Iowa Department of Public Health developed its 1st Five Initiative to address gaps in service provision for young children with risk factors for and evidence of developmental delay during the first years of life (Silow-Carroll, 2008). The program links primary care providers to public health resources and mental and behavioral health services. Features of the program include training primary care providers in assessment of social and emotional development, providing a public health care coordinator to whom the primary care providers could refer children who screened positive, using the coordinator to link the child and family to intervention services, and providing feedback to the primary care provider on the status and outcomes of the referral. This system fostered a coordinated, collaborative approach to care for the developmental needs of at-risk children. Building on its early successes, the initiative had recruited 39 practices serving 41,000 children by 2008 (Silow-Carroll, 2008).

## Organization for Integration

A striking feature that emerged from the literature review is the number of different ways in which integrated efforts were organized. A wide variety of entities were involved in activities and programs that linked primary care and public health. These entities included not only a range of primary care and public health actors but also a number of other contributors, such as businesses, hospitals, academic institutions, and community groups. Additionally, integrated projects were initiated by public health entities, by primary care entities, and by neutral third-party conveners of the two fields, and across examples the extent of the contribution from primary care and public health was varied. Much of this variation is attributable to differences in communities across the country in terms of available primary care, public health, and community resources, as well as in their populations' makeup and health priorities. Successful integration efforts often were tailored to the community's strengths and needs.

A number of examples were initiated and led by public health entities, often health departments. For instance, the health department of

Alachua County, Florida, joined with the local public school system and the University of Florida to initiate a program designed to increase rates of influenza vaccination among school-aged children (Tran et al., 2010). A critical component of the program's success, however, was establishing linkages with primary care providers. Through the vaccination program, children received a free nasal-spray flu vaccine in school, regardless of their insurance status. Children who were ineligible for this vaccine because of underlying medical conditions were referred to their provider for evaluation and the flu shot. This kept private pediatricians in the medical care loop for children with underlying medical conditions, a key component of the medical home concept, as well as a key element in maintaining strong support from community physicians. Both pediatricians and the health department input flu vaccination status into the state's registry so both groups could share information about their patients.[1] In the 3 years since the program became fully operational, immunization rates have increased. In 2009-2010, the program was able to immunize approximately 55 percent of the student population, and an additional 10 percent who could not receive the nasal-spray flu vaccine for medical reasons were immunized by their care providers. In schools where 80 percent or more of the students were eligible for free or reduced-price lunches, the immunization rate went from 12 percent in the 2006 pilot program to 47 percent in 2009-2010 (Tran et al., 2010). Immunization rates for 2010-2011 were similar.[2]

While a majority of the integration examples examined by the committee featured public health-led ventures, there were instances of primary care entities initiating successful collaborations. In Milwaukee, the Sixteenth Street Community Health Center initiated a Community Lead Outreach Project designed to assist in the Milwaukee Health Department's efforts to reduce lead poisoning rates in children by reaching out to an underserved neighborhood. The program employed a team of community outreach workers, led by a nurse-coordinator from the health center. The team conducted home visits, provided blood testing, performed environmental surveys, and reported results to both the health center and the health department for follow-up care and possible intervention. The program resulted in significant decreases in the prevalence of lead poisoning in the area (Schlenker et al., 2001).

In some instances, primary care and public health were brought together by a neutral convener, often a nonprofit organization or academic institution. In the SPARC initiative, discussed previously, a nonprofit organization formed a coalition of primary care, public health, and community groups to take a comprehensive approach to expanding the delivery of

---

[1]Personal communication, C. Tran and Parker Small, University of Florida, November 2011.
[2]Personal Communication, C. Tran, University of Florida, December 2011.

clinical preventive services (Shenson et al., 2008). Organizing the endeavor as a coalition allowed each entity to contribute toward a common goal as befit their respective resources and role in the community.

In North Carolina, the Linkages for Prevention project brought together primary care practices and departments of health in one county to improve health outcomes for low-income mothers and infants (Margolis et al., 2001). The partners formed an advisory board, which included the Medicaid director, community agencies, primary care practices, and county government. The program sought to improve services in both primary care and public health, as well as to enhance communication and coordination of efforts between the two. The program worked to improve the delivery of preventive care in primary care practices and to assist the public health department in implementing intensive home visits to low-income pregnant women and their infants. The home visiting component included conducting two to four visits per month in the infant's first year of life, providing parental education, and linking parents with needed health and human services. To evaluate outcomes, 103 mothers with infants were compared with 105 controls. Improvement was seen in preventive service outcomes, including a higher number of well-child visits by age 12 months (57 percent versus 37 percent), and children were less likely to be seen for injuries and ingestions compared with controls (2 percent versus 7 percent) (Margolis et al., 2001).

## Opportunities for Integration

The literature revealed some promising opportunities for integrating primary care and public health.

**Data** A key opportunity for integrating primary care and public health is sharing data, the focus of a number of examples gleaned from the literature review. Primary care and public health each generate data that can be leveraged by the other to support their respective functions more effectively. Through individual patient visits, primary care generates data that can be used to create population data useful to public health in conducting surveillance or community assessments. Public health assessment data can in turn be tailored to provide valuable information on the health needs and risks of the community served by a particular primary care entity, as well as to allow providers to gauge their clinical performance.

However, several factors hinder sharing data across practices and institutions, including incompatible data systems, varying use of measures, and lack of a trained workforce to develop and implement data sharing strategies. The Indiana Network for Patient Care (INPC) has approached this challenge by creating a united data aggregation hub that receives data from many sources and standardizes them for reuse. While primary care stakeholders and local and state public health organizations are governing members, INPC is separate from primary care and public health systems, and operates by interfacing with these systems and the Indiana community at the data level. INPC is anchored by the Regenstrief Medical Record System, which collects data from a variety of sources, including hospitals, clinics, health departments, and laboratories (McDonald et al., 2005). These data are used to integrate information that can be accessed by providers, researchers, and public health workers participating in the network. A number of provisions ensure that these data are shared safely and appropriately. For clinicians—currently numbering more than 19,000 across the state[3]—INPC provides a community-wide database that enables access to a patient's comprehensive medical record, which includes information that has been generated across multiple sites. The network also receives patient data generated in a wide variety of clinical settings, notifies any of the patient's providers of these reports, and makes the information contained in the reports available to those providers. For public health and research, INPC provides population-based data for epidemiological research and helps identify candidates for particular studies. In addition, it facilitates automated reporting of laboratory results that involve notifiable conditions to state and county health departments. A recent study showed that this automated reporting process helped greatly improve public health efforts in disease surveillance compared with the traditional process of health department notification by clinicians (Overhage et al., 2008).

INPC is an example of an entity separate from primary care and public health acting as a data hub. While the committee's statement of task included exploring the possible role of health departments as data hubs, the INPC model demonstrates the advantages of having a third party administrate such a hub. In this example, the data hub not only provides a health information exchange for use in individual patient services but also is used for population health analyses that serve public health functions. Health information exchanges achieve sustainability by delivering a broad range of cost-effective clinical data services to multiple stakeholder groups across a region or community. Many of these services may not be within the direct purview of traditional public health processes. Thus, while public health may serve as a data hub in some instances, in others it may make more sense for a third party to administer the hub.

**Workforce** Some of the examples from the literature review touch on the need to develop a workforce capable of working in an environment that integrates features and functions of primary care and public health or serv-

---

[3]Personal communication, S. Grannis, Regenstrief Institute, November 2011.

ing as a bridge between primary care and public health activities. In the REACH-Futures program, aimed at reducing infant mortality in inner-city communities in Chicago, registered nurses were teamed with public health–trained community health workers for an infant home-visiting program, managed by a community clinic. The community health workers served to link the clinic's care initiative to public health principles and the community. In the first 4 years of the program, 666 mothers were recruited. Comparison of the REACH-Futures program with a home visiting program using only nurses showed improved retention and immunization rates (Barnes-Boyd et al., 2001).

The George Washington University School of Public Health and Health Services gives its master of public health students a perspective on primary care through its community-oriented primary care (COPC) program (George Washington University School of Public Health and Health Services, 2012). The program is designed to train health and public health professionals in implementing the concept of COPC in practice. As a part of the curriculum, students learn community definition and characterization, problem prioritization, detailed assessment, intervention, and evaluation. As a part of the required practicum, students are expected to work 120 hours in a community setting that offers health services to gain experience in integrating public health initiatives and practices into primary care. To this end, students of this program have participated in practicum experiences covering a wide variety of topics, including hospice care, childhood obesity, community-based rehabilitation, and medication coverage for the elderly.

The Primary Care Leadership Track at Duke University School of Medicine offers emerging physicians a unique opportunity to be trained as leaders capable of engaging the community and to learn various techniques for communicating and practicing to improve health outcomes (Duke University School of Medicine, 2012). Building on partnerships among Duke, the local health department, and the community, the track focuses on matriculating physicians who understand the causes of health disparities, and are driven to create a strong research focus on community engagement and to redesign clinical programs to better meet patient needs at the individual and local population levels. A requirement for the track is a scholarly third year focused on community-engaged research, population studies, or other forms of investigation of health systems and their improvement in collaboration with the Duke Center for Community Research, in partnership with the Durham County Health Department.

## Nongovernmental Public Health

Given the broad nature of public health, a number of organizations, such as academic health centers, research networks, or nonprofit groups, are performing public health functions in various contexts. These organizations can interact meaningfully with primary care to pursue population health improvement, and indeed, many such entities appear in the examples discussed previously as third-party contributors to integration efforts. In areas without a strong governmental public health presence, these organizations can substitute for a health department's role in integration, although they usually are not responsible for the breadth of public health services that a health department typically provides. Some examples from the literature review demonstrate promise for integration but do not fit neatly into the committee's criteria for inclusion; these examples illustrate creative engagement of community resources in addressing community health concerns by working with primary care.

In an effort to better meet the needs of the state's rural population, which suffers from high rates of chronic disease, the University of New Mexico Health Science Center developed the Health Extension Rural Office (HERO) program in 2008 (Kaufman et al., 2010). Modeled after the agricultural extension service, the HERO program engages local agents who live in rural communities in New Mexico and work with the local health system to both foster improvements in the delivery of health services locally and facilitate access to additional services provided by the Health Science Center. These local agents are supported by regional coordinators and Health Science Center staff and work with local partners, including health planning councils, public health clinics, local health clinicians and hospitals, and area health education centers, in each community. The agents work to improve local health services and systems, help recruit a local health care workforce, and strengthen local capacity to address community health problems. In addition to helping secure medical care, HERO agents engage the community to address underlying social issues, such as school retention, food insecurity, and local economic development. They also have trained and deployed community health workers who focus on linking community members to available local resources. These efforts are tightly linked with local primary care providers, and in many cases, the HERO agent also holds a position within the local health care delivery system.

The High Plains Research Network (HPRN) is a community- and practice-based research network located in eastern Colorado. The network engages 16 hospitals/emergency departments, 58 ambulatory clinical practices, and 150 medical providers (University of Colorado, 2008). Housed in the Department of Family Medicine at the University of Colorado School of Medicine, the network is governed by an active Community Advisory Council of rural community members and medical providers (University of Colorado, 2011). The Community Advisory Council comprises 11 community members who live in the High Plains region and includes farmers, ranchers, educators, and retirees. The goal of the Community Advisory

Council is to ground the network's research and programs in the real-life experiences of patients and community members (Van Vorst et al., 2007).

Since its creation in the late 1990s, the HPRN has focused on ameliorating a number of community health problems, including cardiovascular disease, underinsurance, colon cancer, and asthma. Given the high prevalence of asthma (nearly one in six) in the region,[4] the network decided to develop a broad program aimed at increasing knowledge and awareness of asthma and improving the capacity to manage the disease. Led by the Community Advisory Council, the HPRN engaged primary care providers, public health professionals, community members, and university researchers to create two separate asthma toolkits. First, a practice toolkit, which included a spirometer, software, and on-site training, was developed to build capacity in the primary care practices. Two nurse coaches visited every practice, training providers and office staff in evidence-based guidelines for the evaluation and management of asthma and in communication techniques to encourage patient self-management (Bender et al., 2011). Second, a patient toolkit, which included a peak flow meter, an action plan, and culturally relevant educational materials, was developed and distributed to practices for use with asthma patients. Three months after the coaching, practices reported a significant increase in inhaled corticosteroid prescriptions (from 25 percent of practices before the intervention to 50 percent after) (Bender et al., 2011).

## PRINCIPLES FOR SUCCESSFUL INTEGRATION

From the literature review described above, the committee was able to distill a number of principles for successful integration. These principles are listed below and then illustrated through the case studies that follow. The committee believes that to better integrate primary care and public health, the following principles must be in place:

- a shared goal of **population health improvement;**
- **community engagement** in defining and addressing population health needs;
- **aligned leadership** that
  - bridges disciplines, programs, and jurisdictions to reduce fragmentation and foster continuity,
  - clarifies roles and ensures accountability,
  - develops and supports appropriate incentives, and
  - has the capacity to initiate and manage change;

---

[4] Personal communication, J. Westfall, High Plains Research Network, June 2011.

- **sustainability,** key to which is the establishment of a shared infra-structure and a foundation for enduring value and impact; and
- the sharing and collaborative use of **data and analysis.**

## CASE STUDIES

Through its review of the literature, the committee sought examples to use as case studies that demonstrate well-developed relationships between primary care and public health. Rather than highlighting programs designed to manage a single health issue, as is the case for many of the examples discussed previously in this chapter, the committee wanted to showcase linkages between primary care and public health entities that allowed them to join together to overcome a variety of community health challenges. The committee sought such examples that would demonstrate a commitment to an ongoing relationship between the two sectors and reflect the principles for integration outlined above. Case studies from Durham, North Carolina; San Francisco, California; and New York, New York, were selected and are described in this section.

Local communities serve as a laboratory for understanding the prin-ciples underlying successful integration of primary care and public health. The case studies described in this section illustrate how communities across the nation are attempting to bring diverse stakeholders together from the primary care and public health sectors to forge alliances aimed at tackling pressing community health problems and promoting population health. Evaluations of these case studies demonstrate that integration can produce improvements in at least some meaningful measures of system performance and patient-oriented outcomes. However, the case studies are as informa-tive for what they reveal about the process of forging comprehensive and durable cross-sector collaborations as for their outcomes. These examples illustrate innovative practices and important elements of integration that the committee believes are worth highlighting.

### Durham, North Carolina

Durham, North Carolina, is a small city with numerous medical and social resources that have not always translated into improved health outcomes for its inhabitants. Durham's population of 267,000 is about 38 percent African American, 46 percent white (not Latino/Hispanic), and 14 percent Latino/Hispanic (U.S. Census Bureau, 2009), and while the median household income is slightly higher than that for the state of North Caro-lina, Durham residents also experience poverty at a higher than average rate. Furthermore, although Durham possesses a wealth of highly skilled primary care entities, including a top-10 ranked medical school and quickly rising school of nursing (Michener et al., 2008), Durham residents experience rates of chronic disease and health disparity that are only slightly lower than those statewide (Michener et al., 2008). To better align the needs and resources of Durham, a number of partnerships have been created with the assistance of the state and through local determination to improve the health of the city's residents.

## Community Care of North Carolina/Durham Community Health Network

Community Care of North Carolina (CCNC) is an example of a statewide organizational structure developed to coordinate and improve the quality of care for Medicaid recipients through a series of local networks that span the entire state. Guided by a steering committee of primary care physicians, public health professionals, and other stakeholders, CCNC focuses on elements of the patient-centered medical home and chronic care models (Steiner et al., 2008). Although the networks are statewide, each of the 14 local networks is permitted and encouraged to take local actions that build on local strengths and reflect local needs. Each of the networks—including the Durham Community Health Network—is organized and operated by community physicians, hospitals, health departments, and departments of social services under the auspices of the state Medicaid program and with the support of the state medical, hospital, and public health organizations. The networks are funded by small per capita payments from Medicaid, and are responsible for improving outcomes and achieving net savings. The participating primary care practices receive additional per capita payments from Medicaid to support their work toward achieving the network goals.

In Durham, the network is led by a coalition of primary care groups, including the head of the federally qualified health center (FQHC), academic and community primary care practices, the heads of the county departments of health and social services, and the local mental health entity. Locally developed programs include common patient education materials for children with asthma that are used in all health care settings, from school clinics to emergency rooms and specialty practices. A common information technology system is used to track patients and coordinate care management. Programs go beyond the traditional medical model. For instance, the Durham Community Health Network developed the Medicaid In-Home Aide Service. This program uses occupational therapists to conduct home visits to determine whether a personal care assistant is needed, or independent living can be achieved through enhanced behavioral techniques and inexpensive medical devices. From 2008 through 2009, the Medicaid In-Home Aide Service was able to foster independent living for 61 percent of patients requesting aide services, for less than $150 for many individuals (Cook et al., 2010).

## Just for Us

The success of the Durham Community Health Network led to the creation of other coordinated and integrated programs. The Just for Us program is a parallel partnership involving Duke University School of Medicine; Lincoln Community Health Center (an FQHC); the county senior centers; county social, public health, and mental health agencies; and the city housing authority. The program provides coordinated primary care and care management to older adults and adults with disabilities in Durham's public and subsidized housing facilities and group homes. The services are delivered by a multidisciplinary team that includes onsite physician assistants, nurse practitioners, and social workers. Services are supported by Medicaid billings through the FQHC for clinical services and social services provided, and by financial support from Duke Hospital, including payment for social services not reimbursed by Medicaid and funding in recognition of uncompensated emergency room visits avoided (Yaggy et al., 2006). By the end of its second year, Just for Us had expanded to serve nearly 300 patients over 10 locations. The program is demonstrating improvement in individual indexes of health. Medicaid expenditures for enrollees are shifting from ambulance and hospital services to pharmacy, personal care, and outpatient visits (Yaggy et al., 2006).

## Durham Health Innovations

The public health department, community partners, and Duke University School of Medicine collaborated most recently on the Durham Health Innovations (DHI) project to improve health outcomes for the county as a whole. DHI is working in neighborhoods across the county to identify assets for and barriers to care and develop interventions that bring disease prevention, health promotion, and clinical services closer to where citizens live, work, pray, and play. In 2009, DHI funded 10 planning teams charged with developing new methods for reducing morbidity and mortality from diseases identified by the health department as priorities. The 10 teams of community members and clinicians, working with an oversight committee, co-led by the director of public health, and supported by data from the health department and the clinicians' practices, identified seven common elements that could improve health and health care delivery in Durham: (1) increase health care coordination, and eliminate barriers to services and resources; (2) integrate social, medical, and mental health services; (3) expand health-related services provided in group settings; (4) leverage information technology; (5) use "social hubs" such as places of worship, community centers, salons, and barbershops as sites for clinical and social services and information; (6) increase local access to nurse practitioners, physician assistants, and certified nurse midwives; and (7) use traditional marketing methods to influence health behavior (Duke Center for Community Research, 2010).

In 2010, DHI moved into the implementation phase, with the goal of improving health outcomes and access to care for all Durham residents. Current implementation strategies are focusing on two communities identified by the teams and a countywide implementation committee as both ready for change and likely to benefit, and detailed planning for integrated community-based care that connects the residents of these communities to local resources is now under way.

### Principles of Community Engagement

The growing array of programs in Durham involving community groups, the health department, and academic and community physicians led to the establishment of a set of Principles of Community Engagement that includes specific rules for designing and planning such programs, whether clinical, educational, or research oriented (Michener et al., 2005, 2008). The Durham experience highlights the importance of using an approach to integrating primary care and public health centered on the needs of local communities. By coordinating assets through strategic partnerships, Durham leverages existing resources, improves access to and quality of care, and lowers costs.

## San Francisco, California

San Francisco is a city and county with a population of about 800,000, notable for its rich ethnic and cultural diversity. As in most urban areas in the United States, health status varies widely across San Francisco's racial-ethnic and socioeconomic groups and neighborhoods. San Francisco has traditionally had a strong department of public health that is involved extensively in the direct delivery of patient care to uninsured and other vulnerable populations through the operation of San Francisco General Hospital and nearly a dozen FQHCs. The safety net system also includes several unaffiliated HRSA-funded health centers operated as nonprofit organizations. The department of public health has a close relationship with the University of California, San Francisco, in the delivery of patient care, contracting with the university to provide physician staffing at San Francisco General Hospital.

In 2007, San Francisco launched the Healthy San Francisco program to promote universal access to care (Katz and Brigham, 2011) following passage of the San Francisco Worker Health Security Ordinance of 2006. Rather than providing insurance coverage, Healthy San Francisco serves as a structured system for providing uninsured adults with affordable and relatively comprehensive health care services, offered largely at department of public health clinics, San Francisco General Hospital, and federally funded health centers. A cornerstone of the program is linking patients to a primary care medical home. An external evaluation found that Healthy San Francisco was associated with improved access to care, as well as reductions in the use of emergency departments and potentially avoidable hospitalizations (McLaughlin et al., 2011).

Healthy San Francisco has served as an exemplar of a local health department promoting access to health care built on a primary care model; the initiative focuses largely on patient care services rather than on intervention in more upstream determinants of health and illness. The department of public health also is engaged with other stakeholders in broader efforts to integrate primary care and public health to improve population health. One such effort is the San Francisco Health Improvement Partnerships initiative. This initiative originated in 2010 in discussions between leaders in the department of public health and representatives from the National Institutes of Health (NIH)–funded Clinical and Translational Science Institute at the University of California, San Francisco, about how to build more productive collaborations to apply university research assets to solving local public health problems. Diverse constituents in addition to the public health department and the University of California, San Francisco, now participate in the Health Improvement Partnerships, including the San Francisco Hospital Council, the mayor's office, community-based organizations, community clinics, private medical groups and independent physician associations, and the school district. Representatives of many of these constituents serve on a coordinating council, and the Clinical and Translational Science Institute provides staffing and research support to the council and workgroups and pilot funding for the workgroups. Initial projects of the Health Improvement Partnerships are focused on three issues that emerged as priorities from a systematic review of San Francisco health needs assessments, described below.

## High Users of Multiple Services

This project focuses on what have come to be known as "hot spotters" (Gawande, 2011), identifying individuals with extreme social risk factors, such as a combination of homelessness, substance use, and mental illness, that predispose them to unusually high and costly use of emergency, medical, mental health, criminal justice, and related services. The project has created a data warehouse derived from 13 separate databases, which includes data on emergency medical, substance abuse, mental health, medical care, criminal justice, and other services and sectors, to create an individual-level file for each such person. Analyses of these data revealed that the top 10 high-use individuals collectively generated more than $2 million annually in costs for urgent and emergency services alone. The data warehouse is now being used by the department of public health, local Medicaid managed care health plans, and other collaborating agencies to inform strategies for better coordinating services across the primary care, community care, and social services sectors to care for this population more effectively and efficiently.

### Hepatitis B Quality Improvement Collaborative

San Francisco was one of the first cities in the United States to launch a major public health campaign to promote screening for hepatitis B among populations at high risk for chronic hepatitis B. Leaders from the Asian community partnered with the department of public health to develop San Francisco Hep B Free; evaluations have demonstrated the success of this public awareness campaign in increasing screening rates among Asian immigrant populations in San Francisco, about 1 in 10 members of which are chronically infected with hepatitis B (Bailey et al., 2010). The initial public health outreach efforts of Hep B Free led to an appreciation that the primary care clinical system was not adequately prepared to respond to the screening campaign. Initial audits in health department clinics found that many patients were not being screened with the appropriate set of tests and that those testing positive were not consistently receiving follow-up care meeting evidence-based guidelines (Khalili et al., 2010). In response, the initiative developed the Hepatitis B Quality Improvement Collaborative in partnership with Hep B Free and the Health Improvement Partnerships. The Quality Improvement Collaborative has brought together quality improvement leaders from all the major medical groups in San Francisco, including the department of public health, FQHCs, Kaiser Permanente, researchers, and private medical groups, to improve the quality of care in hepatitis B screening and chronic care management for the entire city. One of the first activities has been to share best practices in developing registries of patients with chronic hepatitis B in all the participating medical groups as a cornerstone for more systematic chronic care quality improvement. The collaborative is exploring whether the public health department's mandatory data reporting system for infectious disease surveillance might serve as a substrate for hepatitis B chronic care registries that could be applied in clinical settings by primary care physicians and their medical groups.

*Physical Activity and Healthy Eating*

The Health Improvement Partnerships' work in this area has focused largely on advancing the Shape Up San Francisco campaign, initiated in 2006 by former mayor Gavin Newsom to achieve the population health aim of reducing obesity and chronic disease. An important goal of this work is enhancing coordination of activities across sectors. For example, the Health Improvement Partnerships have facilitated engagement between members of the San Francisco Board of Supervisors and the department of public health, community organizations, and researchers at the University of California, San Francisco, to identify regulatory and tax policies that could be implemented at the local level to promote healthier eating. Other cross-sector projects include Safe Routes to School and facilitation of linkages between primary care clinics and community resources for walking groups, cooking classes, and other wellness activities. These efforts set the stage for the department of public health's successful application for a CDC Community Transformation Grant award in 2011. Interventions under this grant are just starting to be developed, so it is too early to report on specific implementation.

## New York, New York

The most populous city in the United States, New York City provides a unique example of public health in America. Overseeing a city with more than 8 million residents, more than a third of whom are foreign born and nearly 20 percent of whom live below the federal poverty level, the New York City Department of Health and Mental Hygiene (NYC DOHMH) is a local health department with many of the resources and much of the regulatory authority of a state health administration. Over the past decade, many NYC DOHMH programs have embodied the principles of Take Care New York, New York City's comprehensive health policy, which sets goals for population health improvement, generates targeted programs, and monitors their impact and progress toward success (Frieden, 2004). Since the early 2000s, Take Care New York has guided a number of NYC DOHMH initiatives designed to improve the health of city residents. These initiatives focus on the collection and analysis of citywide epidemiological data, the prevention of chronic diseases, and improvements in the social determinants of health. A number of these initiatives have engaged local health care providers and communities.

## Using Electronic Health Records to Support High-Quality Primary Care

In line with the Take Care New York agenda, NYC DOHMH has taken aggressive steps to support high-quality health care and the active management of chronic diseases. At the center of this effort is the Primary Care Information Project, which supports physicians in adopting the use of electronic health records to improve population health. The Primary Care Information Project helped initiate the New York City Regional Electronic Adoption Center for Health (REACH) to assist providers in achieving meaningful use of electronic health records, with the capacity to support 4,500 providers. More than 3,500 providers have already enrolled in REACH to meet the meaningful-use criteria and better serve their communities (NYC Reach, 2011).

To further its promotion of effective use of information technology, NYC DOHMH launched Health eHearts, a pay-for-performance incentive program that rewards small practices and community health centers for achieving excellent heart health among their patients. Designed to reduce health disparities, Health eHearts uses clinical quality outcomes generated from electronic health records and provides incentives up to $25,000 per quarter to practices showing qualifying improvements in the use of aspirin, blood pressure and cholesterol management, and the promotion of smoking cessation to improve cardiovascular health. By the end of 2010, 42 practices had received an average of $38,000 each for their efforts in these areas (Marcello et al., 2011). Also in 2010, NYC DOHMH launched the Panel Management Program to help primary care providers maintain continuity of care for high-risk patients and those with chronic disease. Using registry features of electronic health records, prevention outreach specialists identify patients who are at risk for diseases associated with hypertension, high cholesterol, smoking, and diabetes, and then contact them with reminders about disease management activities such as making appointments, filling prescriptions, and receiving vaccinations (New York City Department of Health and Mental Hygiene, 2011).

## Monitoring and Surveillance

The Panel Management Program's capacity for monitoring and evaluation is grounded in the Community Health Survey, which regularly surveys 10,000 New York City residents to gather data on a variety of health measures. In 2004, a community-level Health and Nutrition Examination Survey was conducted, modeled after the nationwide survey conducted by CDC. The data thus collected resulted in several publications released by NYC DOHMH, including *Health Bulletin*, which directs its public health messages to city residents (Frieden et al., 2008). In addition, NYC

DOHMH was one of the first local health departments to implement syndromic surveillance—the routine surveillance of health care encounters to detect public health threats—in part to address the threat of a potential bioterrorist attack. NYC DOHMH has partnered with health care facilities to implement systems that provide its staff with nonconfidential data for daily analysis aimed at identifying disease trends and outbreaks by scanning for clustering by symptoms or health care-seeking behavior. NYC DOHMH currently monitors visits to 48 city emergency departments. Every day, hospitals transmit an electronic file to NYC DOHMH containing patients' chief complaint, age, sex, zip code, and time of visit. The chief complaint is automatically coded as one of four syndromes (respiratory, fever-flu, vomiting, or diarrhea), and standardized analyses are performed 7 days a week by a corps of analysts at NYC DOHMH. Syndromic surveillance has enhanced the ability of public health to monitor community illness in a way that is timelier, though less specific, than traditional surveillance based on laboratory or provider reports (Heffernan et al., 2004).

## Community Outreach

NYC DOHMH actively engages with local communities to promote health education and access to care. It is participating in two home visiting programs for new mothers. One of these programs, the Nurse-Family Partnership, aligns nurses with first-time mothers for weekly to biweekly visits until the child is 2 years old (Nurse-Family Partnership, 2011). The second program, the Newborn Home Visiting Program, is localized to Brooklyn, Harlem, and the Bronx. A health worker attempts to visit every new mother to promote health education, breastfeeding, and the reduction of environmental risks in the home.

NYC DOHMH also conducts community outreach to promote cancer screening. In 2003, it established the Colonoscopy Patient Navigator Program to ensure that populations facing greater screening obstacles receive a colonoscopy. The navigators are tasked with helping patients navigate the health system and overcome barriers to screening. By 2007, the Colonoscopy Patient Navigator Program had assisted more than 25,000 New Yorkers in undergoing colonoscopies. Through this program and other initiatives of Take Care New York, NYC DOHMH has seen remarkable gains in cancer screening, attributable mainly to its ability to partner with local care providers and communities. Overall rates of colon cancer screening have increased substantially since the introduction of Take Care New York—by 43 percent from 2002 to 2006; by 2009, 66 percent of adults over age 50 had been screened for colon cancer within the previous 10 years (Frieden et al., 2008; Marcello et al., 2011).

## Principles of Integration Embedded in the Case Studies

The case studies described here illustrate the principles, presented earlier, that form the foundation for integrating primary care and public health.

Each of these case studies exemplifies a shared goal of **population health improvement**. This goal was realized in different ways in different locations. In New York, for example, the department of public health took the initiative, but only through joint efforts with primary care providers were improved outcomes possible. In San Francisco, collaborative efforts built on the success of Healthy San Francisco as a health access innovation, and then evolved to embrace a broader vision of population health.

The case studies have been presented within the context of their local communities because one unifying theme is the local variability seen in sustainable examples of integration. **Community engagement** is required throughout the process. In San Francisco, the community was engaged in diverse ways—not only through the traditional primary care and public health sectors but also through community-based social service organizations, political leaders, and academic researchers. Community Care of North Carolina offers a statewide organizational structure, but provides for flexibility for each of the 14 local networks to take action based on local strengths and needs. In Durham, for example, community engagement guided integration efforts using an approach that recognizes and draws on the strengths of the local community.

The third principle, **aligned leadership,** is embodied in each of these case studies. Aligned leadership involves more than directing a program. It reflects the ability to bridge disciplines, programs, and jurisdictions, as in the case of Durham's Just for Us, a partnership among a community health center, county social and mental health agencies, an academic health center, and a city housing authority. Aligned leadership also entails the ability to clarify roles and ensure accountability. Community Care of North Carolina reflects the development of incentives to encourage integration. The networks created through this partnership are funded by small per capita payments based on the achievement of improved outcomes and net savings. Primary care practices receive additional per capita payments to support their population health activities. Similarly, the public health department in New York City works with primary care providers to promote cardiovascular health by providing financial incentives. Developing and supporting appropriate incentives is another aspect of leadership. The final element of aligned leadership is the capacity to initiate and manage change. In moving from the status quo to an innovative approach, each of these examples reflects this element.

Making a commitment to **sustainability** is the fourth principle. This commitment to sustainability is illustrated by San Francisco, where resources were pooled, and by Community Care of North Carolina, where dedicated funding streams ensure that the program will have an enduring value and an enduring impact.

Finally, integration requires that **data and analyses** be shared and used collaboratively. Integration of data has been central to the work in San Francisco, from linking data sets on high users of multiple services, to agreeing on uniform hepatitis B quality metrics, to identifying existing data sources with which to track progress on physical activity and healthy eating.

While the committee believes that all these principles are ultimately necessary to integrate and sustain integration efforts, it also believes that integration can start with any of these principles and that starting is more important than waiting until all the elements are in place.

## HOW THE EXAMPLES AND CASE STUDIES ILLUSTRATE EFFECTIVE PRIMARY CARE AND PUBLIC HEALTH INTEGRATION

The committee's statement of task included identifying examples for a number of aspects of effective primary care and public health integration. Rather than identify a separate programmatic example for each aspect, however, the committee approached this task by looking for programs that illustrate multiple aspects. Table 2-3 highlights the examples and case studies that relate to each aspect identified in the statement of task.

## LESSONS LEARNED

The literature review provided many valuable lessons about the state of primary care and public health integration. First, it highlighted that there are a wide variety of such activities taking place in communities throughout the United States. These activities embody many different approaches to integration, reflecting the needs of the local community, the available local resources, and the local partners that are willing and able to come together. This emphasis on local differences means there is no generalizable solution to integration that the committee can propose. However, the many impressive local efforts can influence action at the federal level.

The importance and difficulty of achieving sustainability is another lesson. Many of the partnerships described in the literature were short term, funded by grants and either decreasing in scope or disappearing altogether when the source of external funding dried up. Embedding integration activities in existing structures to ensure that they continue after external funding has stopped is key to sustaining these activities. Sustainability continues to challenge local partners and has limited the impact of successful primary care and public health integration efforts in the past.

**TABLE 2-3** Aspects of Primary Care and Public Health Integration
Illustrated by the Examples and Case Studies

| Aspect | Examples |
| --- | --- |
| Demonstrated, shared accountability for population health improvement | Evident in all of the examples, this aspect is especially illustrated by the **Community Care North Carolina** networks. These networks are led by local physicians, public health officials, and other stakeholders who meet to discuss local health trends and establish statewide priorities for health. Once established, these priorities are taken back to the local community, where local workers determine how the desired result in a given priority area will be achieved. |
| Optimizing the integration of the public health and primary care workforce | The **George Washington University School of Public Health and Health Services** provides its master of public health students with a primary care perspective through its community-oriented primary care (COPC) program. As part of the required practicum, COPC students are expected to work 120 hours in a community setting that offers health services to gain experience in integrating public health initiatives and practices into primary care. To this end, students have participated in practicum experiences covering a wide variety of topics, including hospice care, childhood obesity, community-based rehabilitation, and medication coverage for the elderly. |
| Collaborative governance | The **San Francisco Health Improvement Partnerships** highlight the effectiveness of collaborative governance. The Coordinating Council for the partnerships includes leaders from the primary care and public health sectors, along with many community stakeholders. The diversity of participants in the decision-making process allows for a more comprehensive evaluation of community health challenges and innovative solutions. |
| Collaborative financing | Embedded in **Community Care North Carolina** is a collaborative financing structure in which primary care payments from Medicaid are used in conjunction with public health funding streams to support joint community-level activities, including the coordination of care. |

**TABLE 2-3** Continued

| Aspect | Examples |
|---|---|
| Collaborative care coordination models | **Community Care North Carolina** has a focus on the coordination of care and services through its locally managed networks, drawing on the patient-centered medical home and chronic care models. One example is the Just for Us program in Durham, which highlights coordinated primary care and care management for older adults and adults with disabilities in Durham's public and subsidized housing facilities and group homes. |
| Effective use of health information technology, including | The **Indiana Network for Patient Care (INPC)** is an example of the effective use of health information technology. The system collects data from hospitals, clinics, laboratories, and physicians within the network and uses these data to populate and maintain patient records, to notify local and state departments of public health of laboratory results, and to provide a wealth of epidemiologic data to researchers and public health officials. |
|   • Reporting of notifiable conditions | **INPC's** automated notifications system is an example of the use of health information technology to report the occurrence of notifiable conditions. This system has greatly improved surveillance and reporting of such conditions in Indiana. |
|   • Coordination on care and follow-up to improve outcomes | **New York City** provides a valuable example of using health information technology to coordinate care and follow-up to improve outcomes. The Panel Management Program uses prevention outreach specialists to identify patients at high risk of diabetes, high cholesterol, hypertension, and smoking by means of electronic health records and contacts these patients to encourage positive behaviors such as filling prescriptions, making and keeping follow-up appointments, and receiving vaccinations. |

*continued*

**TABLE 2-3 Continued**

| Aspect | Examples |
|---|---|
| • Primary care systems and public health departments as potential hubs | The **New York City Department of Health and Mental Hygiene** provides an example of innovative data collection and analysis performed within a public health department. **INPC**, on the other hand, illustrates a centralized, stakeholder-governed data storage and analysis system that operates independently of primary care and public health systems. The data are controlled by their providers, who are members of the primary care and public health communities; under contract with INPC, they allow some data to be isolated and aggregated with data gathered from other members to create a clearer image of population health. These aggregate data can be accessed by INPC members at the discretion of the owners for the purposes of clinical evaluation, population surveillance, or clinical research. |
| • Sentinel surveillance systems | **New York City** uses a syndromic sentinel surveillance system as an early warning system for disease outbreaks. This system requires electronic reporting from emergency departments and ambulance services within 24 hours for encounters involving certain flu-like and gastrointestinal symptoms. It also requires pharmacies to report sales of relevant over-the-counter and prescription medications to public health officials. |
| • Progress on exchanging electronic health record generated information | **INPC** shows excellent progress on the standardization and dissemination of the information collected from network members. These data are available to provide comprehensive individual health records to network physicians and public health officials, as well as population-based data for epidemiological research. |

Related to sustainability is the difficulty of achieving scalability. Integration activities in local communities rarely are able to move beyond their initial start-up site. There are some exceptions, including SPARC and the case studies. Overall, however, scalability is a challenge in promoting integration.

One of the positive lessons is that sharing data and a workforce appears to be a natural way in which primary care and public health can work together. In all of the case studies and many of the examples, sharing data to address community health concerns was foundational for integration efforts. Similarly, the possibility of sharing staff as a way to bring primary care and public health together was a frequent theme in the literature.

## ROLE OF HRSA AND CDC

The examples and case studies provide some glimpses of HRSA and CDC involvement: the Community Transformation Grant awarded to San Francisco; health centers involved in various communities; and HRSA's provision of funding to Regenstrief Institute, Indiana State Department of Health, and the Public Health Informatics Institute to develop guidance for better management of child health (Grannis et al., 2010). However, the agencies were not the genesis of the integration; the integration was already happening at the local level. As mentioned above, the committee believes there are some ways in which HRSA and CDC could make a greater contribution to these processes.

At a minimum, recognition of the overlapping contributions of the two agencies would be helpful. Whether it be prenatal care; childhood immunization campaigns; prevention, tracking, and treatment of sexually transmitted diseases; cardiovascular disease; or cancer, the work of the two agencies is bound together at the level of the community. But separate project requirements, data systems, and administrative structures complicate the coordination of needed services. Coordinated planning between the agencies would assist communities in linking their programs to serve their clientele better and more efficiently.

Coordination would assist in reducing the tensions that can exist with respect to which community agency "owns" an issue or program. Which agency or group is leading locally depends on local history and relationships. Allowing variation in structure while requiring the achievement of common goals would permit building on local strengths and successes and reduce unnecessary tensions.

More broadly, coordination between the agencies could create a space in which others could participate. Improving population health is a task requiring both agencies, but is larger than both combined. Private and academic medical practices, hospitals, schools, social services, mental health agencies, parks and recreation, and community groups all have perspectives, strengths, and resources to contribute. Several of the examples and case studies described in this chapter demonstrate the value of an initial primary care–public health partnership that expands to include others.

Similarly, the coordination of data collection and tracking would assist local efforts. If health departments and HRSA-supported health centers were tracking the same data and if these data were available locally, the data would provide a common understanding of opportunities for the community and a way in which stakeholders could gauge their performance in meeting community needs.

Another point that emerges from the literature is the need to develop the human capital required for integration. Bridging disciplines is not easy in the best of times and is much more challenging when there are major stressors and uneven talent and skills. Fundamental shifts are necessary in the training of both primary care and public health practitioners so they can work together effectively in meeting the needs of their communities.

The examples and case studies also demonstrate that what is needed is less support for initial integration, although that is still helpful, and more the removal of barriers that impede the development and expansion of integration activities that are already taking place at the local level.

Finally, HRSA and CDC could assist in evaluating local integration efforts. This would help create a more robust evidence base with associated health and process outcomes. This evidence base, in turn, could illuminate potential benefits and best practices or methods for integration.

## REFERENCES

Bailey, M. B., R. Shiau, J. Zola, S. E. Fernyak, T. Fang, S. K. S. So, and E. T. Chang. 2010. San Francisco Hep B Free: A grassroots community coalition to prevent hepatitis B and liver cancer. *Journal of Community Health* 36(4):538-551.

Barnes-Boyd, C., K. Fordham Norr, and K. W. Nacion. 2001. Promoting infant health through home visiting by a nurse-managed community worker team. *Public Health Nursing* 18(4):225-235.

Bender, B. G., P. Dickinson, A. Rankin, F. S. Wamboldt, L. Zittleman, and J. M. Westfall. 2011. The Colorado asthma toolkit program: A practice coaching intervention from the High Plains Research Network. *The Journal of the American Board of Family Medicine* 24(3):240-248.

Constance, A., K. Crawford, J. Hare, S. Parker, A. Scott, A. Stys, and G. May-Aldrich. 2002. MDON: A network of community partnerships. *Family & Community Health* 25(3):52-60.

Cook, J., J. L. Michener, M. Lyn, D. Lobach, and F. Johnson. 2010. Community collaboration to improve care and reduce health disparities. *Health Affairs* 29(5):956-958.

Duke Center for Community Research. 2010. *Durham health innovations.* https://www.dtmi. duke.edu/about-us/organization/duke-center-for-community-research/durham-health-innovations (accessed November 15, 2011).

Duke University School of Medicine. 2012. *Duke primary care leadership track.* http://duke-med.duke.edu/modules/ooa_myedu/index.php?id=35 (accessed January 23, 2012).

Frieden, T. 2004. Take Care New York: A focused health policy. *Journal of Urban Health* 81(3):314-316.

Frieden, T. R., M. T. Bassett, L. E. Thorpe, and T. A. Farley. 2008. Public health in New York City, 2002-2007: Confronting epidemics of the modern era. *International Journal of Epidemiology* 37(5):966-977.

Gawande, A. 2011. Hot spotters. *The New Yorker*, January 24.

George Washington University School of Public Health and Health Services. No Date. *Community-oriented primary care.* http://www.gwu.edu/learn/graduateprofessional/finda graduateprogram/fulllistofprograms/communityorientedprimarycare (accessed January 23, 2012).

Grannis, S., B. Dixon, and B. Brand. 2010. *Leveraging immunization data in the e-health era: Exploring the value, tradeoffs, and future directions of immunization data exchange.* Indianapolis, IN: Public Health Informatics Institute and Regenstrief Institute.

Heffernan, R., F. Mostahari, D. Das, A. Karpati, M. Kulldorff, and D. Weiss. 2004. Syndromic surveillance in public health practice. *Emerging Infectious Diseases* 10(5):858-864.

Katz, M. H., and T. M. Brigham. 2011. Transforming a traditional safety net into a coordinated care system: Lessons from healthy San Francisco. *Health Affairs* 30(2):237-245.

Kaufman, A., W. Powell, C. Alfero, M. Pacheco, H. Silverblatt, J. Anastasoff, F. Ronquillo, K. Lucero, E. Corriveau, B. Vanleit, D. Alverson, and A. Scott. 2010. Health extension in New Mexico: An academic health center and the social determinants of disease. *Annals of Family Medicine* 8(1):73-81.

Khalili, M., J. Guy, A. Yu, A. Li, N. Diamond-Smith, S. Stewart, M. Chen, and T. Nguyen. 2010. Hepatitis B and hepatocellular carcinoma screening among Asian Americans: Survey of safety net healthcare providers. *Digestive Diseases and Sciences* 56(5):1516-1523.

Larson, K., J. Levy, M. G. Rome, T. D. Matte, L. D. Silver, and T. R. Frieden. 2006. Public health detailing: A strategy to improve the delivery of clinical preventive services in New York City. *Public Health Reports* 121(16640143):228-234.

Lasker, R. D., and the Committee on Medicine and Public Health. 1997. *Medicine and public health: The power of collaboration.* New York: The New York Academy of Medicine.

Marcello, R. K., C. Mortezazadeh, C. Chang, and T. Farley. 2011. *Take Care New York 2012; tracking the city's progress 2009-2010.* New York: New York City Department of Health and Mental Hygiene.

Margolis, P. A., R. Stevens, W. C. Bordley, J. Stuart, C. Harlan, L. Keyes-Elstein, and S. Wisseh. 2001. From concept to application: The impact of a community-wide intervention to improve the delivery of preventive services to children. *Pediatrics* 108(11533360): E42.

Martin-Misener, R., R. Valaitis, and The Strengthening Public Health Care Through Primary Care and Public Health Collaboration Research Team. 2009. *A scoping literature review of collaboration between primary care and public health: A report to the Canadian Health Services Research Foundation.* Hamilton, ON: StrengthenPHC.

McDonald, C. J., J. M. Overhage, M. Barnes, G. Schadow, L. Blevins, P. R. Dexter, and B. Mamlin. 2005. The Indiana network for patient care: A working local health information infrastructure. An example of a working infrastructure collaboration that links data from five health systems and hundreds of millions of entries. *Health Affairs* 24(5):1214-1220.

McLaughlin, C., M. Colby, E. Taylor, M. Harrington, T. Higgins, V. Byrd, and L. Felland. 2011. *Evaluation of Healthy San Francisco.* Ann Arbor, MI: Mathematica Policy Research.

Michener, J. L., M. T. Champagne, D. Yaggy, S. D. Yaggy, and K. M. Krause. 2005. Making a home in the community for the academic medical center. *Academic Medicine* 80(15618094):57-61.

Michener, J. L., S. Yaggy, M. Lyn, S. Warburton, M. Champagne, M. Black, M. Cuffe, R. Califf, C. Gilliss, R. S. Williams, and V. J. Dzau. 2008. Improving the health of the community: Duke's experience with community engagement. *Academic Medicine* 83(4): 408-413.

New York City Department of Health and Mental Hygiene. 2011. *Primary care information project.* http://www.nyc.gov/html/doh/html/pcip/panel-management.shtml (accessed December 2011).

Nurse-Family Partnership. 2011. *Public funding: A sound investment that can yield substantial public and private gains.* Denver, CO: Nurse-Family Partnership.

NYC Reach. 2011. *NYC Regional Extension Center for Health IT.* http://www.nycreach.org/ (accessed December 2011).

Overhage, J. M., S. Grannis, and C. J. McDonald. 2008. A comparison of the completeness and timeliness of automated electronic laboratory reporting and spontaneous reporting of notifiable conditions. *American Journal of Public Health* 98(2):344-350.

Rothemich, S. F., S. H. Woolf, R. E. Johnson, K. J. Devers, S. K. Flores, P. Villars, V. Rabius, and T. McAfee. 2010. Promoting primary care smoking-cessation support with quitlines: The QuitLink randomized controlled trial. *American Journal of Preventive Medicine* 38(4):367-374.

Schlenker, T. L., R. Baxmann, P. McAvoy, J. Bartkowski, and A. Murphy. 2001. Primary prevention of childhood lead poisoning through community outreach. *Wisconsin Medical Journal* 100(8):48-54.

Shenson, D., W. Benson, and A. C. Harris. 2008. Expanding the delivery of clinical preventive services through community collaboration: The SPARC model. *Preventing Chronic Disease* 5(1):A20.

Silow-Carroll, S. 2008. Iowa's 1st Five Initiative: Improving early childhood developmental services through public-private partnerships. *Issue Brief (Commonwealth Fund)* 47:1-15.

Sloane, P. D., J. Bates, M. Gadon, C. Irmiter, and K. Donahue. 2009. *Effective clinical partnerships between primary care medical practices and public health agencies.* Chicago, IL: American Medical Association.

Steiner, B. D., A. C. Denham, E. Ashkin, W. P. Newton, T. Wroth, and L. A. Dobson, Jr. 2008. Community care of North Carolina: Improving care through community health networks. *Annals of Family Medicine* 6(4):361-367.

Tran, C. H., J. McElrath, P. Hughes, K. Ryan, J. Munden, J. B. Castleman, J. Johnson, R. Doty, D. R. McKay, J. Stringfellow, R. A. Holmes, P. D. Myers, P. A. Small, and J. G. Morris. 2010. Implementing a community-supported school-based influenza immunization program. *Biosecurity and Bioterrorism: Biodefense Strategy, Practice, and Science* 8(4):331-341.

University of Colorado. 2008. *About HPRN.* http://www.ucdenver.edu/academics/colleges/medicalschool/departments/familymed/research/PBRN/HPRN/Pages/AboutHPRN.aspx (accessed November 12, 2011).

University of Colorado. 2011. *The Anschutz medical campus.* http://www.ucdenver.edu/about/denver/ Pages/AnschutzMedicalCampus.aspx (accessed December 14, 2011).

U.S. Census Bureau. 2009. Estimates of the resident population by race and hispanic origin for the United States and states: July 1, 2008 (SC-EST2008-04). Washington, DC: U.S. Census Bureau.

Van Vorst, R. F., R. Araya-Guerra, M. Felzien, D. Fernald, N. Elder, C. Duclos, and J. M. Westfall. 2007. Rural community members' perceptions of harm from medical mistakes: A High Plains Research Network (HPRN) study. *The Journal of the American Board of Family Medicine* 20(2):135-143.

Yaggy, S. D., J. L. Michener, D. Yaggy, M. T. Champagne, M. Silberberg, M. Lyn, F. Johnson, and K. S. H. Yarnall. 2006. Just for Us: An academic medical center-community partnership to maintain the health of a frail low-income senior population. *The Gerontologist* 46(2):271-276.

# 3

# Potential for Interagency Collaboration

In response to its statement of task, the committee examined how primary care systems supported by the Health Resources and Services Administration (HRSA) and public health departments supported by the Centers for Disease Control and Prevention (CDC) could integrate in specific areas. (Descriptions of HRSA-supported primary care systems and state and local health departments can be found in Appendix B.) The term "health center" is used here to refer to organizations that receive grants under the Health Center Program as authorized under section 330 of the Public Health Service Act, as amended, and federally qualified health center look-alike organizations, which meet all the Health Center Program requirements but do not receive Health Center Program grants. The term does not refer to federally qualified health centers that are sponsored by tribal or urban Indian health organizations, except for those that receive Health Center Program grants.

The committee selected three areas on which to focus: maternal and child health (MCH) (specifically the Maternal, Infant, and Early Childhood Home Visiting Program), cardiovascular disease prevention, and colorectal cancer screening. These topics were selected because they lend themselves to a life-course perspective, involve aspects of mental and behavioral health, and touch on issues relevant to health disparities. They also represent a mix of programs led by HRSA and CDC.

The principles presented in Chapter 2 were used as an organizing framework for the discussion of these three areas. The discussion of each area is organized in two parts: (1) how the area relates to the principles, and (2) potential actions, needs, or barriers that affect primary care–public health integration in the area.

## MATERNAL AND CHILD HEALTH

One of the provisions of the Patient Protection and Affordable Care Act (ACA) creates the Maternal, Infant, and Early Childhood Home Visiting Program (referred to here as the Home Visiting Program). While the term "home visiting" can have different meanings in different contexts, it generally refers to a trained professional who visits a new mother in her home to provide advice and support and assess the home environment for the newborn. This provision of the ACA is based on years of work suggesting that home visiting for at-risk families can prevent child abuse and neglect, promote child development, increase parental support and effectiveness, and assist in reducing health disparities (Chapman et al., 1990; Duggan et al., 2000; Olds et al., 1997, 2004). In 2009, the American Academy of Pediatrics endorsed home visiting as an early-intervention strategy that benefits children, and encouraged the development of comprehensive programs that target at-risk families and involve professionally trained home visitors (AAP, 2009).

The aim of the grant-based Home Visiting Program is to go beyond individual patient care to include care for families that live in high-risk communities. Nurses, social workers, or other trained professionals visit at-risk families in their homes and connect them to health care or other services, such as early education, child abuse prevention, or nutrition assistance. The law requires that states conduct statewide needs assessments to identify at-risk communities, defined as communities with high concentrations of certain types of health risks among children, adolescents, and families. State assessments also must determine the quality of existing programs and their capacity to carry out home visiting and consider the gaps that exist in such programs. Based on the results of these assessments, the Department of Health and Human Services (HHS) is directed to make grants to early childhood home visiting programs to promote improvements in health and socioeconomic status and reduce community and family risks.

The Home Visiting Program represents a strong opportunity for integration of primary care and public health because the health care service delivered is not based on an illness or in response to a person seeking care, but instead is aimed at prevention and wellness for all members of a community. This program is administered by HRSA in collaboration with the Administration for Children and Families (ACF), but could be strengthened through collaboration with CDC. The following section examines the Home Visiting Program according to the principles of integration outlined in Chapter 2 and highlights opportunities for HRSA and CDC.

## Principles of Integration

*Shared Goal of Population Health Improvement*

The benchmarks for the Home Visiting Program are broad, encompassing areas that touch on the social determinants of health, such as a family's economic self-sufficiency and improvement in school readiness and achievement. Box 3-1 provides a list of all six benchmark areas.

By including the family and community as targets of interest, the program embraces an ecological perspective on health. Thus, the program was designed from a population health point of view and begins with the goal of improving population health. To make this a shared goal of HRSA and CDC, CDC could be involved in extending the program's reach.

*Community Engagement*

The Home Visiting Program was designed to engage the community with a two-fold emphasis on families who need services and the communities in which those families reside. The grant application requires a detailed needs and resources assessment of a targeted community and specifies the selection of a home visiting program that responds directly to the community's identified needs. Linking at-risk families to local health centers strengthens (or in some cases creates) a relationship between primary care providers and the family. Through the conduct of rigorous evaluations, key lessons can be distilled that will allow programs to be replicated, recognizing that each community will require a slightly different implementation.

---

**BOX 3-1
Benchmark Areas for the Maternal, Infant, and
Early Childhood Home Visiting Program**

- Improved maternal and newborn health
- Prevention of child injuries; child abuse, neglect, or maltreatment; and reduction of emergency department visits
- Improvement in school readiness and achievement
- Reduction in crime or domestic violence
- Improvements in family economic self-sufficiency
- Improvements in coordination and referrals for other community resources and supports

SOURCE: *Patient Protection and Affordable Care Act of 2010 (ACA)*, Public Law 148, 111th Cong., 2d sess. § 2951 (March 23, 2010).

---

Through its work with the Community Transformation Grants,[1] CDC is well positioned to be involved in supporting community engagement in the Home Visiting Program. HRSA and CDC could investigate ways in which these two community-based programs could interface. Linkages could be explored between communities selected for Home Visiting Program grants and those selected for Community Transformation capacity-building grants. For example, groups that received grants from CDC to disseminate and amplify lessons learned from Community Transformation Grant programs could work with HRSA to include strategies learned from the Home Visiting Program.

### Aligned Leadership

The Home Visiting Program emphasizes key relationships and opportunities for creating aligned leadership. At the federal level, cooperation with the ACF is required; this requirement has been extended to include the Department of Education, the Department of Justice, the Assistant Secretary of Policy and Evaluation at HHS, and others (Yowell, 2011). At the state level, the grant application requires sign-off by a number of agencies, such as the state child welfare agency, the Child Care and Development Fund, and the State Advisory Council on Early Childhood Education and Care authorized by the Head Start Act. Merely signing off on a document does not indicate aligned leadership, but it does create an opportunity for building a relationship that could lead to alignment. At the local level, the needs assessment process built into the program encourages the forging of local relationships, thereby offering opportunities for relationship building among MCH providers, community health workers,[2] community-based organizations, and other critical stakeholders. Each of these opportunities presents an occasion for bridging disciplines, clarifying roles, initiating and managing change, and developing appropriate incentives.

Other opportunities exist to build aligned relationships. For example, HRSA currently has 22 staff persons dedicated to the Home Visiting Program. This includes a dedicated Home Visiting Program staff person as well as a dedicated staff person for the Title V State Block Grant program at each of the 10 regional HHS offices. This co-location in each of the regional HHS offices fosters on-the-ground collaboration and integration of these

---

[1] Community Transformation Grants were authorized in the ACA. For more detailed information, see Chapter 4.

[2] A community health worker is defined as a person who links members of the community to health services. The designation encompasses *promotores de salud* (community health workers in Spanish) and patient navigators (who work with specific patients), as well as other terms.

MCH programs within HRSA. Currently, CDC has no MCH staff in these offices. Building relationships between HRSA and CDC staff at the regional level would help align priorities and the implementation of MCH activities. At the state level, the requirement for a needs assessment provides an opportunity for health departments to work with implementing partners. Finally, as programs mature and are evaluated, health departments and implementing partners will have an opportunity to coalesce around strong programs and advocate for the adoption and dissemination of promising results.

*Sustainability*

As part of the Home Visiting Program, states must create a resource plan and discuss how the program will fit into existing programs within the community. These actions contribute to the program's sustainability. On the other hand, it is important to note that the program is funded for only 5 years. Its survival depends on converting its elements into a sustainable practice and financing model, which means building interest and engagement on the part of state Medicaid programs, the overwhelming source of health care financing in the highest-risk communities. In fostering this engagement, HRSA and CDC could educate payers, namely the Centers for Medicare & Medicaid Services (CMS) and state Medicaid programs, on the health and financial effects of home visiting, particularly those that allow state programs to begin to reduce costs. Specifically, they could encourage CMS to track the children and families involved in this program to assess its effectiveness.

One of the stated goals of the Home Visiting Program is to "establish home visiting as a key early childhood service delivery strategy in high-quality, *comprehensive* statewide early childhood systems [emphasis in original]" (Yowell, 2011, p. 7). Given the importance of health across the life course, home visiting is an excellent starting point to support the health of young children; however, its impact depends on linkages to other services for children and families, such as early childhood programs; the Special Supplemental Nutrition Program for Women, Infants, and Children (WIC); and Head Start. Beyond conducting a needs assessment, the program could require demonstrating that these links are in place to better serve the target population.

Furthermore, through its Maternal and Child Health Epidemiology Program, CDC, in collaboration with HRSA, is working to build capacity in the area of MCH epidemiology. This program assigns senior epidemiologists to state public health departments, as well as local health departments and other venues, in an effort to build analytical capacity focused on the health of women and children. The state needs assessments required by the Home Visiting Program provide an opportunity to work closely with state health departments, and the Maternal and Child Health Epidemiology Program could be used as a bridge between the two entities.

## Data and Analysis

Data collection is a fundamental component of the MCH work undertaken by both HRSA and CDC. Through its Title V block grant program, HRSA requires that states and jurisdictions report annually on national performance measures, health system capacity indicators, national outcome measures, and health status indicators. In addition, each state develops 7 to 10 state performance measures to address identified priorities and unique needs not addressed by the national measures. Healthy Start, another program administered by HRSA's Bureau on Maternal and Child Health, requires that grant recipients report data on the characteristics of their program participants, as well as the services they provide. Finally, data collection is a core component of the Home Visiting Program. States must submit a plan that demonstrates how data will be collected for each of the benchmark areas listed earlier in Box 3-1.

At CDC, the Pregnancy Risk Assessment Monitoring System (PRAMS) is an ongoing state- and population-based surveillance system designed to collect information on self-reported maternal behaviors and experiences that occur around the time of pregnancy. This data collection effort generates statewide estimates of perinatal health indicators among women who recently delivered a live infant. Each participating state uses a standardized data collection method developed by CDC. PRAMS staff in each state collect data through mail and telephone questionnaires. Because PRAMS data are state and population based, findings are generalizable to an entire state's population of women delivering a live-born infant. PRAMS not only solicits information concerning the timing of and barriers to obtaining prenatal care, but also assesses knowledge, attitudes, and behaviors to identify strengths and shortcomings of current models of prenatal care. Similarly, the National Vital Statistics System, part of CDC's National Center for Health Statistics, collects information about the timing of the onset of prenatal care. When combined with the number of prenatal visits, this information can be used to assess the adequacy of prenatal care (Heaman et al., 2008).

With the wealth of MCH data being collected, the opportunity for promoting integration is strong. In fact, in some ways cooperation is already taking place. For example, CDC's PRAMS serves as a data source for HRSA's Title V activities. And both agencies have moved to make their data sources more accessible. CPONDER is a web-based program that allows users to access data from PRAMS, while the Title V Information System provides access to Title V data. Progress has been made toward allowing researchers and the public more access to each agency's data sets, and some of the data are informing programs in other agencies. However, there has been no real move to coordinate the data to maximize efficiencies and assist the end users. The Home Visiting Program offers numerous opportunities for HRSA and CDC to collaborate in establishing practice and outcome performance measurements, but better integration of their data systems will be necessary if these opportunities are to be exploited.

### Potential Actions, Needs, and Barriers

The Home Visiting Program represents a move toward a population health approach. However, integration with CDC could strengthen the program and its impact. HRSA and CDC could take action in the following areas to achieve a partnership based in the Home Visiting Program.

*Finance*

Although financing for the Home Visiting Program has been ensured for 5 years, HRSA and CDC need to plan for the program's sustainability. One action that could be taken to this end would be to work with state Medicaid directors to gather evidence about the financial benefits of this program by tracking the children who are involved. Having this information would give state Medicaid directors an understanding of the benefits of the program and its value to their Medicaid populations. Incorporating the Home Visiting Program would challenge the notion of what services Medicaid considers to be within its funding scope. Medicaid will pay for services that involve personal health care, including behavioral health and child development services by home visitors. However, it traditionally has not paid for a home visitor to spend time on community health issues or on coordination with such entities as social service agencies, housing services, and WIC; these are deemed to be public or community health services not focused on individual patients, and therefore not reimbursable. The Home Visiting Program provides HRSA and CDC with an opportunity to reposition the discussion about funding and promote population health by working with state Medicaid directors to sustain this program.

Currently, MCH programs are funded by HRSA and CDC through separate funding streams, which can create barriers at the local level. There is a need to support local integration efforts by coordinating funding streams at the agency level, thereby empowering primary care providers and public health departments to work together at the local level.

## Governance

HRSA and CDC need to provide aligned leadership in the area of governance. The two agencies could consider first establishing their own partnership and then developing training programs in leadership for state and local primary care providers and public health workers. This training could encourage the development of broad community partnerships focused on complex MCH problems.

## Health Information Technology

Increased data sharing and concrete movement toward the integration of health information technology are needed. A sustained effort on the part of HRSA and CDC to promote data sharing among existing Title V, PRAMS, Healthy Start, and other MCH programs administered by HRSA and CDC would strengthen these programs. In addition, the two agencies could advance efforts to improve data sharing and service development in local communities by jointly leading efforts to establish pathways for integration of health information technology with other federal agencies, such as the U.S. Department of Agriculture, which oversees the WIC program. Such integration would facilitate tracking and measuring community-level data that can inform the development of community interventions. For example, understanding the migration patterns in and out of a community; the age distribution of the population; the availability and condition of housing stock; and how all of these and related factors affect children, mothers, and families would make it possible to devise more effective interventions.

## Delivery System and Practice

CDC's expertise in MCH currently is not represented in HHS's regional offices. Providing a staff person who could work directly with the MCH staff provided by HRSA in the regional offices offers an opportunity to align goals around MCH. In addition, directly involving local health centers in the Home Visiting Program would foster relationships between primary care providers and families. And creating and maintaining linkages between the Home Visiting Program and other services for children and families would ensure continuity. HRSA could require such linkages as a formal part of the program.

Finally, by linking the Home Visiting Program with data provided by CDC, HRSA could use the program to focus its attention on emerging at-risk communities before they become truly at risk. CDC could train state health departments to determine at-risk or emerging at-risk communities and then use those skills to feed into the statewide needs assessment required by the Home Visiting Program.

## Workforce Education and Training

A potential way to expand the capacity of the local workforce would be to conduct training for primary care providers and state and local public health workers in community needs assessments that take advantage of existing data and incorporate assessment of local resources beyond health care. Examples of such resources include transportation, food availability, and the capacity to partner with social and educational service providers. HRSA and CDC could work together to provide this training.

## CARDIOVASCULAR DISEASE PREVENTION

The American Heart Association estimates that approximately 82.6 million people have one or more forms of cardiovascular disease (Roger et al., 2011). Common forms of cardiovascular disease include coronary heart disease, hypertension (high blood pressure), stroke, and heart failure. In 2007, more than 813,000 people died from a cardiovascular disease—more than from cancer, chronic lower respiratory disease, and accidents combined. As the leading cause of death, coronary heart disease was responsible for nearly half of these deaths (406,351). More than 150,000 of these individuals were younger than 65 years of age. Cardiovascular disease also is an important example of health disparities. African Americans experience significantly higher mortality rates from cardiovascular disease than whites: in 2007, the overall cardiovascular disease death rate per 100,000 was 251.2; the rate was 405.9 and 286.1 for African American males and females, respectively, versus 294.0 and 205.7 for their white counterparts. And death is not the only outcome of cardiovascular disease. As of 2007, approximately 7 million Americans aged 20 and older had experienced a stroke, a leading cause of disability in the United States (Roger et al., 2011).

Cardiovascular disease also is very expensive. In 2007, it was estimated to cost more than $286 billion, including $167 billion in direct costs associated with physicians and other health professionals, in-patient services, medications, etc., and $119 billion in indirect costs resulting from lost productivity, illness, and death (Roger et al., 2011).

To combat cardiovascular disease, specifically heart attacks and strokes, a joint effort involving HHS, other government agencies, and private-sector partners was launched in September 2011 (Frieden and Berwick, 2011). Known as the Million Hearts initiative, this effort has the goal of preventing 1 million heart attacks and strokes over the course of 5 years. While this effort clearly extends beyond HRSA and CDC working together, the committee believes that, given its size and its recent launch, this initiative is the best example with which to illustrate how collaboration between the two agencies around the topic of cardiovascular disease prevention could be strengthened. CDC, along with CMS, is the lead agency for this initiative. Many other agencies, including HRSA, are listed as partners, and all bring an impressive list of programs to bear.

As part of the Million Hearts initiative, HRSA and CDC have committed to some integrated activities that are worth noting. Specifically, HRSA is developing new measures for health center program grantees to track aspirin use and drug therapy for lowering LDL cholesterol (HRSA, 2012). If these measures are approved, beginning in 2012, health centers will be required to report annually on them, in addition to the current measures that track blood pressure control and smoking cessation. Known collectively as ABCS, aspirin use, blood pressure control, cholesterol management, and smoking cessation are four key areas CDC emphasizes as ways to prevent heart attacks and strokes (CDC, 2010). By linking these areas to health center program grantee reporting, the agencies will be aligning behind a common goal.

There are other programmatic areas in which HRSA and CDC are working to prevent heart attacks and strokes. Linking these programs together, where appropriate, could strengthen each agency's contribution to the achievement of the Million Hearts goal.

## Principles of Integration

### Shared Goal of Population Health Improvement

The Million Hearts initiative suggests that the HHS agencies have a shared goal of population health improvement. Achieving the reduction in strokes and heart attacks targeted by the initiative—which is a population health goal—will require contributions from all of the agencies involved. No one agency, regardless of how effectively its programs are run, can reach the targeted goal by working alone.

One program HRSA oversees that is contributing to this effort is the Healthy Weight Collaborative, which aims to encourage healthy weight and health equity. This program, funded by HRSA and administered by the National Initiative on Children's Healthcare Quality, works with health care delivery, public health, and community-based organizations (HRSA and National Initiative for Children's Health Care Quality, 2011). In its first phase, the collaborative established a team from each HRSA region (10 teams in all) composed of representatives from all three of these sectors (HRSA and National Initiative for Children's Health Care Quality, 2011). The collaborative is a public–private partnership that involves numerous stakeholders. It embraces a population health approach by recognizing that obesity is a multifaceted problem that must be addressed by many parties working together.

CDC's Community Transformation Grants are another example of a population health-focused program aimed at reducing the burden of chronic disease in communities by addressing heart disease, stroke, and other diseases. CDC is using these grants to further the goals of the Million Hearts initiative by giving priority to grantees that work to address cardiovascular risk factors. The population health focus of the Healthy Weight Collaborative and the Community Transformation Grants could be a starting point for exploring ways in which HRSA and CDC could work together toward their shared goal of population health improvement. While the two programs use different approaches, involving CDC in the Healthy Weight Collaborative and involving HRSA in the Community Transformation Grants could strengthen each program by building on the knowledge each has acquired.

*Community Engagement*

In addition to the Healthy Weight Collaborative and the Community Transformation Grants, the portfolios of HRSA and CDC include other programs that involve local communities in the prevention of cardiovascular disease. For example, CDC's Division for Heart Disease and Stroke Prevention administers the WISEWOMAN program, which focuses on reducing the burden of cardiovascular disease among women aged 40 to 64 who are financially disadvantaged. While adhering to a common set of parameters, the program is implemented differently depending on the circumstances of the individual community, but includes such activities as promoting healthy cooking, walking, and smoking cessation. Additionally, through a demonstration project that was recently expanded, HRSA supports community health workers who assist patients with chronic disease, including cardiovascular disease. These community health workers have different tasks based on the needs of the patient population in their community, but they frequently encourage healthy behaviors, assist patients in navigating complex health care systems, and inform members of the community about appropriate screenings. Similarly, CDC's Division for Heart Disease and Stroke Prevention works in 41 states and the District of Columbia to increase state capacity to define the local burden of cardiovascular disease and design culturally appropriate interventions to address the problem.

With HRSA and CDC each engaging local communities in the effort to promote cardiovascular health, the challenge is getting these programs to work together. Using the Million Hearts initiative as an opportunity, HRSA and CDC could explore ways in which their programs could leverage each other to better support community engagement. One clear opportunity is around the sharing of lessons learned. For example, health centers are at the forefront of confronting disparities in health care. A major health disparity is that some communities are disproportionately impacted by hypertension and heart attacks (IOM, 2010). Many of these communities are served by health centers. Thus, the experience of health centers with successful strategies to achieve better outcomes in blood pressure and cholesterol control could be used to advise the WISEWOMAN program and Community Transformation Grants. In many cases, health centers have been pioneers in employing culturally relevant outreach and educational methodologies and bilingual modalities that could be used more effectively in public health activities aimed at cardiovascular disease prevention. Having HRSA and CDC facilitate the sharing of these lessons would strengthen their programs.

### Aligned Leadership

HHS should be recognized for its leadership in bringing multiple programs and agencies together to take on the challenge of reducing strokes and heart attacks. In a key area related to the prevention of cardiovascular disease, HHS also has demonstrated leadership by developing an action plan for combating tobacco use. This plan encompasses a comprehensive inventory of all HHS agencies and programs related to tobacco use (HHS, 2010), as well as working groups that also involve numerous agencies, including HRSA and CDC. However, leadership could be expanded to bridge disciplines and reduce fragmentation. Leadership also has a role in ensuring accountability and developing the appropriate incentives to encourage the implementation of strategies and the achievement of health targets.

In the case of the Million Hearts initiative, the leadership of HHS could do more to encourage the various agencies involved to work together toward the reduction of heart attacks and strokes. And by stating that they will work together to accomplish the goals of Million Hearts, leaders of HRSA and CDC would be sending a powerful message that collaboration will take them farther down the road of preventing a million heart attacks and strokes than either agency could go on its own. Likewise, the leadership of HRSA and CDC could work to promote partnerships between the two agencies' programs.

### Sustainability

Individual programs tied into the Million Hearts initiative may work toward sustainability. For example, by including measures that track tobacco use and body mass index, HRSA already has moved to embed cardiovascular disease prevention in health centers. Similarly, CDC's WISE-WOMAN program encourages communities to make enduring changes by addressing the risk factors for heart disease and stroke.

Beyond the contributions of these individual programs, there is an opportunity to build linkages between programs to create a solid infrastructure that could be sustained to address cardiovascular disease. While the Million Hearts initiative will be in place for 5 years, the challenge will be to create an enduring infrastructure that will continue beyond this initiative's lifetime. This could be accomplished by leveraging the strengths of HRSA and CDC. For example, health centers are primed to demonstrate the outcome of clinical interventions in a relatively short time frame. In other words, HRSA's commitment to gathering data on cholesterol management, blood pressure control, and aspirin use can be shown, within a relatively short time, to result in a decrease in cardiovascular events. On the other hand, CDC's Community Transformation Grants focus on interventions that rely on community engagement and education. These interventions hold promise for yielding outcomes that will be observed within a longer time frame, such as a decrease in adults with a diagnosis of prediabetes or hypertension. Linking the components of HRSA's work with the components supported by CDC could lead to sustainable improvements in population health. By working jointly on the Million Hearts initiative, the two agencies could create the opportunity to engage patients in behaviors and medication therapy at the primary care level while at the same time promoting broader public health and community messages and activities. Conversely, public health outreach could connect community members to primary care and individualized therapy.

*Data and Analysis*

As suggested earlier, data from primary care sources can inform public health and population health efforts. For instance, data from clinical settings could be combined with geographic data to create maps illustrating the burden of disease by neighborhood. These maps could be used by primary care providers as well as public health professionals. Thus, to take one example, patterns of diabetes and poor control of the disease could be displayed on maps that could direct shared primary care and public health resources. These maps could then be tracked over time, making visible the efficacy of integrated primary care and public health efforts. Since health centers are identified largely as providing care for medically underserved areas, mapping patterns of clinical efficacy against Community Transformation Grants and other CDC efforts should promote collaborative activity and accountability.

In addition, linking existing data sets overseen by HRSA and CDC would facilitate integration efforts related to cardiovascular disease. The Uniform Data System (UDS) collects a variety of data from health centers, including patient demographics, clinical services, and services provided. As mentioned above, new measures have been proposed to capture data on aspirin use and drug therapy for cholesterol management. Annual UDS data are available to researchers and the public through HRSA's website. CDC has developed the National Cardiovascular Disease Surveillance System, which combines multiple data sets to provide a comprehensive picture of the public health burden of heart disease. An interactive website has been designed to display these data and make them user-friendly (CDC, 2011b). Collectively, these two data systems contain a wealth of information, but they currently must be accessed separately. Linking these systems would provide a detailed view of cardiovascular health at the local, state, and national levels.

## Potential Actions, Needs, and Barriers

The Million Hearts initiative offers HRSA and CDC a unique opportunity to align their cardiovascular disease prevention efforts more closely. This process could begin with action in the following areas.

### Science

Many HRSA and CDC programs currently under way are focused on preventing cardiovascular disease. A potential action that would build on these programs would be to evaluate their effectiveness and share the lessons learned from those evaluations with the other agency. Those lessons could assist the other agency in designing future programs focused on cardiovascular health, as well as highlight some areas in which integration could be fostered.

### Finance

HRSA and CDC could provide some flexibility for grantees that are pursuing the goals of the Million Hearts initiative. For example, the agencies could permit some grantees to set requirements around screening or outreach that would give health departments and health centers added flexibility in their fight against cardiovascular disease.

### Governance

The leadership of HRSA and CDC could commit to aligning their programs within the Million Hearts initiative. The two agencies could use the opportunity of this larger effort to foster a spirit of collaboration that would permeate the agencies and encourage collaborative efforts at the program level.

## Health Information Technology

Currently, HRSA and CDC have separate databases that hold information on cardiovascular health at the local, state, and national levels. While each of these databases is accessible to the public, they need to be coordinated to provide a comprehensive picture of the population's health with respect to cardiovascular disease. HRSA and CDC could develop new and perhaps standardized databases for joint use. They also could jointly create and utilize maps and geographic data that would reflect the health status of the population and highlight areas of greatest need. This would allow HRSA and CDC to combine efforts in those locations and direct the use of shared resources.

## Delivery System and Practice

HRSA and CDC could align around each of their strengths to improve integration in the area of delivery system and practice. CDC's public education campaigns on cardiovascular health could be focused in areas with HRSA-supported health centers. The campaigns could include messages encouraging people to seek care at health centers. Also, building on evidence showing that primary care providers play a key role in encouraging their patients to stop smoking (Valery et al., 2008), providers at health centers could partner with local and state health departments that are implementing tobacco cessation programs.

## Workforce Education and Training

HRSA and CDC could use the National Health Service Corps (NHSC) and the Epidemic Intelligence Service (EIS) to work together in communities to prevent cardiovascular disease. As primary care providers working with underserved populations, officers of the NHSC are well positioned to provide clinical services, including those that promote cardiovascular health, to vulnerable community members. EIS officers based in state and local health departments likewise are well positioned to use public health approaches to address cardiovascular disease. The desire to improve the health of communities unites these programs. By working together, their workforces could make significant contributions to the prevention of cardiovascular disease in underserved populations.

## COLORECTAL CANCER SCREENING

Colorectal cancer is the third most commonly diagnosed cancer and third leading cause of death due to cancer for both men and women (American Cancer Society, 2011). The American Cancer Society estimates that in 2012, colorectal cancer will be responsible for approximately 9 percent of all cancer deaths (American Cancer Society, 2012); for 2011, it is estimated that 141,210 people were diagnosed with colorectal cancer, and 49,380 died from the disease (American Cancer Society, 2011). CDC has reported that from 2003 to 2007, the incidence of colorectal cancer decreased from 52.3 per 100,000 population to 45.5 per 100,000 and that the mortality rate decreased from 19 to 16.7 per 100,000—a decline of 66,000 cases and 32,000 deaths compared with 2002. According to CDC, "screening prevented approximately half of the expected new [colorectal cancer] cases and deaths during 2003-2007 (33,000 new cases and 16,000 deaths)" (CDC, 2011c, p. 889). For screening for colorectal cancer, the U.S. Preventive Services Task Force recommends use of the high-sensitivity fecal occult blood test (FOBT), sigmoidoscopy with FOBT, or colonoscopy, which carry a Grade A recommendation for all people aged 50 to 75 (U.S. Preventive Services Task Force, 2008). Yet despite the proven effectiveness of screening, approximately 22 million individuals have never been screened for colorectal cancer (CDC, 2011c).

Unfortunately, significant disparities exist in the colorectal cancer screening rates for a number of populations. In 2008, CDC (2011a) found that only 51.2 percent of Hispanics and 62.9 percent of African Americans and Asian and Pacific Islanders over age 50 were up to date on routine colorectal cancer screening, compared with 66.2 percent of whites. Furthermore, only 48.6 percent of those with less than a high school diploma and 49.4 percent of those earning less than $15,000 had been appropriately screened, compared with 72.1 percent of college graduates and 74.8 of those earning at least $75,000 in the same age group. CDC also found that while 66.6 percent of insured individuals over age 50 had received routine screening, this was the case for only 37.5 percent of those without insurance (CDC, 2011a).

CDC's Colorectal Cancer Control Program funds colorectal cancer control activities in 25 states and 4 tribes. The program, which provides funding for a total of 5 years, has two components—screening promotion and screening provision. Each component is carried out by the states and tribes. The screening promotion component is based on evidence-based strategies recommended by the Task Force on Community Preventive Services and adapted to local situations. Screening and follow-up care are provided to low-income adults aged 50-64 who are unable to pay. The program encourages offering the screening in collaboration with other publicly funded health programs or clinics.

Another CDC program, Screen for Life, is an educational campaign that uses celebrities to encourage older adults to get screened for colorectal cancer. The program has been in existence since 1999. Educational materials for patients and health care providers have been developed in conjunction with the program's outreach campaign,

While HRSA does not have a colorectal cancer program, integrating CDC's ongoing colorectal cancer screening activities with the patient-centered medical home transformation process now being initiated at HRSA-supported health centers would appear to be a good way to reach populations with traditionally low colorectal cancer screening rates. In a move to strengthen colorectal cancer screening, HRSA has proposed a new clinical quality performance measure for health centers that, if approved, will track colorectal cancer screening for adults aged 50 to 75.

Finally beyond HRSA and CDC, a number of other HHS agencies have cancer screening programs. HRSA and CDC should consider including these agencies in their partnerships.

## Principles of Integration

### Shared Goal of Population Health Improvement

CDC's Colorectal Cancer Control Program was designed to address economic disparities by providing screening for those who would not otherwise be able to obtain it. This emphasis on vulnerable populations aligns with the work of health centers, which serve these populations. By formally encouraging states participating in the Colorectal Cancer Control Program to link to local providers, CDC is building on this strength of health centers. Several states have made these links. And by including the new proposed performance measure on colorectal cancer screening, HRSA has positioned health centers to work with health departments in identifying members of the population who should be screened.

### Community Engagement

The states and tribes receiving funding from CDC's Colorectal Cancer Control Program tailor their screening promotion activities to their local environment. Drawing on strategies that have been evaluated by the Task Force on Community Preventive Services ensures that promotion activities are grounded in evidence, but the program allows them to be adapted to the specific conditions in recipient states and tribes.

One way health centers connect with the local environment is through the use of patient navigators. Patient navigators come from the populations they serve and assist community members with the screening process. With colorectal cancer screening, the tasks they undertake can vary from outreach to communities at homes, places of worship, shopping malls, or places of employment to inreach into medical records to determine who needs to be screened. Once screening has been accepted by patients, the tasks undertaken can be as simple as getting patients to return FOBT tests or arranging a colonoscopy for patients with a positive test. Paskett and colleagues (2011) report that patient navigators spent an average 2.5 hours per case assisting patients. The most common barriers for these patients were (1) out-of-pocket expenses, (2) transportation, and (3) fear of having and dealing with a positive test. Early findings from HRSA's Patient Navigator Outreach and Chronic Prevention Demonstration Program show that 76 percent of the program's patients referred to primary care followed up on that referral, and 68 percent of patients referred for screening services made an appointment (Peplinski et al., 2011). The enormous potential of patient navigators or other community health workers to link the community to health centers is documented in several studies that show significant increases in colorectal cancer screening rates (Jandorf et al., 2005; Percac-Lima et al., 2008).

While primary care and public health both are engaging the community to combat colorectal cancer, there is no formal link between them. Requiring a needs assessment as part of the Colorectal Cancer Control Program to identify activities already taking place in the state—similar to the needs assessment required by the Home Visiting Program discussed above—would enable states to identify and link with primary care delivery sites, such as health centers, early on. Similarly, encouraging states and tribes to use patient navigators who can link patients to health centers would create an opportunity for partnership.

*Aligned Leadership*

Much of CDC's work on colorectal cancer has been built on the success of the National Breast and Cervical Cancer Education Program. This program, which began in 1991, has forged many relationships among providers, public health workers, and others. Building on this foundation through the Colorectal Cancer Control Program gives CDC the opportunity to leverage these existing relationships, clarifying roles and ensuring accountability. These are key aspects of aligned leadership.

A number of groups share the goal of increasing colorectal cancer screening. In addition to health centers, which have strong relationships in the communities in which they work, these groups include state cancer plans, primary care associations, state public health associations, medical societies, national cancer centers, and others. No one group can combat colorectal cancer alone. Coordinating these groups and aligning their leadership would ensure an integrated approach to colorectal cancer screening. One opportunity for encouraging this coordination is the National Colorectal Cancer Roundtable, which includes representatives of federal agencies, advocacy groups, medical groups, and other interested parties. Rather than create a new structure for aligning leadership in this area, HRSA and CDC could work with the roundtable to encourage coordination.

*Sustainability*

Funding for the Colorectal Cancer Control Program is available until 2014. The 25 states and 4 tribes selected for this 5-year program frequently run their colorectal cancer screening activities through the state health department, although this is not always the case. Embedding colorectal cancer activities in an existing cancer control program or the state health department will help sustain the program. To have a lasting impact on the incidence of colorectal cancer, however, the delivery of screening services also must be sustainable.

With the proposed colorectal cancer screening measure, providers at health centers may have an added incentive to provide screening; if approved, this measure will require them to report their screening rates. Screening rates should be bolstered by the finding of the U.S. Preventive Services Task Force that colorectal cancer screening is a Grade A recommendation for those aged 50 to 75 and thus will be covered by all insurance expansion under the ACA. Bringing health centers into the Colorectal Cancer Control Program's activities should provide a sustainable venue for the delivery of screening services.

Continuity is particularly important in the context of a screening program. If colorectal cancer incidence rates are to be reduced, not only must individuals be screened, but in some cases follow-up care with a specialist outside of a health center also will be required. For an enduring impact, relationships must be established and roles clarified. CDC could contribute to meeting this need by requiring that continuity be addressed as part of its Colorectal Cancer Control Program. And HRSA could require that continuity be an integral part of the patient-centered medical home model being adopted by health centers.

*Data and Analysis*

Health centers collect and report performance measures through the UDS, which allows them to track their screening rates. As noted above, a new measure on colorectal cancer screening has been proposed and, if approved, will be added next year. This could serve to focus health centers on their screening rates. Health center records (either paper or electronic) could become a significant source of data on population screening rates. Some health centers are already using electronic health records, and these records will serve as a mechanism for collecting data on colorectal cancer at the patient level and reporting them to health departments. However, most electronic health records currently are incapable of tracking and reporting population-level data. The development of electronic health records that can track population-level data and the adoption of this technology by health centers should be encouraged.

CDC already has created a system for reporting breast cancer screening and outcome data that could be expanded for colorectal cancer. As with cardiovascular disease prevention, the coordination of these two data systems is key to integrating activities in colorectal cancer screening.

## Potential Actions, Needs, and Barriers

CDC is well positioned to assist health centers in meeting the needs of their at-risk populations. Other groups, such as the Colorectal Cancer Roundtable (of which CDC was a founding member), primary care associations, and others can contribute to the work of health centers in increasing the colorectal cancer screening rates of their service populations. Thus, relationships designed to promote colorectal cancer screening should involve not only health centers, health departments, HRSA, and CDC, but also other interested groups. The actions outlined below could be taken by HRSA and CDC to integrate their efforts in colorectal cancer screening.

### Finance

One barrier related to finance is that CDC's funding for the Colorectal Cancer Control Program will end in 2014. There is a need to embed this program's activities in state health departments or other entities to ensure that the activities will be sustained after the funding ends. Some states have been successful in doing this. CDC should encourage all participating states to move in this direction. As part of the effort to make the program an integral part of state health departments, formal links should be forged with health centers to ensure access to screenings.

### Health Information Technology

Opportunities abound for health centers and health departments to share data related to colorectal cancer screening; however, there are some unmet needs and barriers to realizing these opportunities. Specifically, health centers need to be able to track population-level data so it is clear who has been screened and who has not. Health centers and health departments also need to be able to share data on colorectal cancer screening. Currently, there is little coordination between HRSA and CDC with respect to their databases, and this lack of coordination acts as a barrier to integration. The two agencies could coordinate their databases and work jointly to develop new data sets in the future.

## Policy

A potential action that would go a long way toward reducing the incidence of colorectal cancer would be to engage advocacy groups in urging congressional action on coverage for the costs of colorectal cancer treatment. Congress has given states the option to cover breast and cervical cancer treatment through Medicaid, and this model could be applied to colorectal cancer. As noted, with the coverage expansion to take place under the ACA, screening for colorectal cancer will be covered for those aged 50 to 75 because it has received a Grade A recommendation from the U.S. Preventive Services Task Force for this age group. Congressional action giving states the option to use Medicaid to cover the cost of treatment would enable continuity of care for those with a positive screening.

## Workforce Education and Training

Strengthening the role of patient navigators is a potential action in the area of workforce education and training. Patient navigators offer an opportunity for integration by linking the community to primary care. These positions could be funded either by health centers or by health departments (or jointly). Another potential action is the creation of materials to inform and support the workforce with respect to colorectal cancer screening. A good example is the toolkit created in North Carolina with the involvement of numerous stakeholders (Rohweder et al., 2011).

## OPPORTUNITIES FOR INTERAGENCY COLLABORATION

In its review of the three areas discussed in this chapter, the committee was struck by both the vastly different organizational structures of HRSA and CDC, which create logistical barriers to the formation of partnerships, and, despite these barriers, the willingness of the two agencies to work together.

HRSA is organized into bureaus and operational offices, with each bureau being organized around an aspect of clinical service delivery. Therefore, it is not surprising that HRSA has neither a cardiovascular disease program nor a colorectal cancer program (although it does have a Maternal and Child Health Bureau). On the other hand, CDC is organized around diseases and health topics. This structure naturally lends itself to programs on MCH, cardiovascular disease, and colorectal cancer. These structural differences mean there often is no natural link between the agencies. This situation is not necessarily negative. In fact, like puzzle pieces that fit into place, these structural differences can actually further the overall goal of better coordination. Ideally, the two agencies could work in concert with health centers providing care to individuals identified through a CDC program as having a disease-specific condition but also in need of other care. In the short run, however, the differences can mean that staff from one agency do not always have a natural counterpart in the other.

Yet staff from HRSA and CDC do appear to be willing to partner, as do the agencies' leaders. While jointly sponsoring this report is one indication of this willingness, there are others. In November 2009, for example, HRSA and CDC staff held a 3-day meeting to develop an agenda for working more collaboratively (HRSA, 2010). In October 2011, the two agencies jointly organized a Primary Care/Public Health Forum in Macon, Georgia. The meeting was an opportunity for those working in HRSA-supported primary care clinics and in health departments to become aware of their colleagues' work and discuss how they could coordinate in the future. And staff of both agencies were generous with their time in meeting with the committee to discuss the three areas covered in this chapter.

From the committee's in-depth examination of the Home Visiting Program, cardiovascular disease prevention, and colorectal cancer screening, some key points emerged. They include the value of using community health workers, the opportunities provided by data sharing, the potential to use the NHSC and the EIS to create linkages in communities, and the possibility of using a third party to foster integration.

Community health workers, including *promotores de salud* and patient navigators, fill a unique space between primary care practice and public health. As members of the community, they are an integral part of the population and can advance public health initiatives by linking community members to personalized care. They appear to enhance efforts focused on the prevention of cardiovascular disease and colorectal cancer screening and can be used in home visiting programs. In addition, HRSA's Patient Navigator Outreach and Chronic Disease Prevention Demonstration Program is showing some preliminary positive outcomes (Peplinski et al., 2011). The role of community health workers thus appears to be an element of the workforce discussion that should be further explored and expanded.

Opportunities related to data sharing are evident in all three areas. HRSA and CDC collect and analyze large amounts of data, and coordinating these data efforts is a clear means of promoting integration. Finding a way to achieve this coordination for specific topics such as MCH would leverage the contributions of each agency while strengthening the overall field, and could provide important benefits to communities and the end users of these databases. One concern is that as data systems move forward, they will not be developed in a way that allows primary care providers to communicate with health departments. HRSA and CDC should work with the Office of the National Coordinator at HHS to encourage health centers and health departments to adopt systems with consistent standards and technology. It is also critical that local communities have access to these data to better understand the health status of the local population and inform policy. CDC, in particular, could play a role in facilitating this access by encouraging state health departments to involve local health departments and health centers in the design of surveillance systems, data hubs, and other data collection activities.

The NHSC and the EIS, respectively, are HRSA's and CDC's primary workforce programs. The section on cardiovascular disease prevention addresses how these two programs could be engaged jointly to prevent cardiovascular disease, but this joint engagement could occur in any area. With NHSC and EIS officers being situated in communities throughout the country, the potential to combine forces to benefit local populations is significant. By harmonizing these programs, HRSA and CDC could expand the reach of both programs and assist in integration at the community level.

Finally, using a third party appears to be a successful strategy for encouraging collaborative efforts. The third party could be an outside group, such as the National Colorectal Cancer Roundtable or the Institute of Medicine, that would bring HRSA and CDC staff together physically around a topic. Alternatively, the third party could be a policy structure such as the National Prevention Strategy, the National Quality Strategy, or the Million Hearts initiative. Such a third party appears to act as a catalyst, encouraging collaboration that might not happen otherwise. For example, HRSA and CDC are working together on the Tobacco Control Strategic Action Plan. Without this plan as a mechanism for sharing information and aligning programs, this collaboration might not be seen as a priority. Staff at both agencies are busy, and finding the time to work together often requires a compelling reason, such as reporting on an initiative. As the two agencies work toward greater collaboration, they may want to seek out opportunities for third parties to bring them together.

## REFERENCES

AAP (American Academy of Pediatrics). 2009. The role of preschool home-visiting programs in improving children's developmental and health outcomes. *Pediatrics* 123(2):598-603.

American Cancer Society. 2011. *Colorectal cancer facts and figures 2011-2013*. Atlanta, GA: American Cancer Society.

American Cancer Society. 2012. *Cancer facts & figures 2012*. Atlanta, GA: American Cancer Society.

CDC (Centers for Disease Control and Prevention). 2010. *Strategies for states to address the "ABCS" of heart disease and stroke prevention*. Atlanta, GA: CDC.

CDC. 2011a. Colorectal cancer screening—United States, 2002, 2004, 2006, and 2008. *Morbidity and Mortality Weekly Reports* 60(01):42-46.

CDC. 2011b. *Division for heart disease and stroke prevention: Data trends & maps*. http://apps.nccd.cdc.gov/NCVDSS_DTM/ (accessed December 15, 2011).

CDC. 2011c. Vital signs: Colorectal cancer screening, incidence, and mortality—United States, 2002–2010. *Morbidity and Mortality Weekly Reports* 60(26):884-889.

Chapman, J., E. Siegel, and A. Cross. 1990. Home visitors and child health: Analysis of selected programs. *Pediatrics* 85(6):1059-1068.

Duggan, A., A. Windham, E. McFarlane, L. Fuddy, C. Rohde, S. Buchbinder, and C. Sia. 2000. Hawaii's healthy start program of home visiting for at-risk families: Evaluation of family identification, family engagement, and service delivery. *Pediatrics* 105(Suppl. 2):250-259.

Frieden, T. R., and D. M. Berwick. 2011. The "Million Hearts" initiative—preventing heart attacks and strokes. *New England Journal of Medicine* 365(13):e27.

Heaman, M. I., C. V. Newburn-Cook, C. G. Green, L. J. Elliott, and M. E. Helewa. 2008. Inadequate prenatal care and its association with adverse pregnancy outcomes: A comparison of indices. *BMC Pregnancy and Childbirth* 8(1):15.

HHS (Department of Health and Human Services). 2010. *Ending the tobacco epidemic: A tobacco control strategic action plan for the U.S. Department of Health and Human Services*. Washington, DC: Office of the Assistant Secretary for Health.

HRSA (Health Resources and Services Administration). 2010. *Public Health Steering Committee recommendations: Reinvigorating HRSA's public health agenda*. Washington, DC: HRSA.

HRSA. 2012. *Proposed uniform data system changes for 2012 program assistance letter 2012-01*. http://bphc.hrsa.gov/policiesregulations/policies/pal201201.html (accessed January 15, 2012).

HRSA and National Initiative for Children's Health Care Quality. 2011. *Collaborate for healthy weight*. http://www.collaborateforhealthyweight.org/About.aspx (accessed December 15, 2011).

IOM (Institute of Medicine). 2010. *A population-based policy and systems change approach to prevent and control hypertension*. Washington, DC: The National Academies Press.

Jandorf, L., Y. Gutierrez, J. Lopez, J. Christie, and S. H. Itzkowitz. 2005. Use of a patient navigator to increase colorectal cancer screening in an urban neighborhood health clinic. *Journal of Urban Health: Bulletin of the New York Academy of Medicine* 82(2):216-224.

Olds, D. L., J. Eckenrode, C. R. Henderson, H. Kitzman, J. Powers, R. Cole, K. Sidora, P. Morris, L. M. Pettitt, and D. Luckey. 1997. Long-term effects of home visitation on maternal life course and child abuse and neglect—fifteen-year follow-up of a randomized trial. *Journal of the American Medical Association* 278(8):637-643.

Olds, D. L., H. Kitzman, R. Cole, J. Robinson, K. Sidora, D. W. Luckey, C. R. Henderson, C. Hanks, J. Bondy, and J. Holmberg. 2004. Effects of nurse home-visiting on maternal life course and child development: Age 6 follow-up results of a randomized trial. *Pediatrics* 114(6):1550-1559.

Paskett, E. D., J. P. Harrop, and K. J. Wells. 2011. Patient navigation: An update on the state of the science. *CA: A Cancer Journal for Clinicians* 61(4):237-249.

Peplinski, K., C. McLeod, and D. Stark. 2011. Use of patient navigators as a strategy to increase access to care for health disparities populations. Paper read at APHA 139th Annual Meeting and Exposition, Washington, DC.

Percac-Lima, S., R. W. Grant, A. R. Green, J. M. Ashburner, G. Gamba, S. Oo, J. M. Richter, and S. J. Atlas. 2008. A culturally tailored navigator program for colorectal cancer screening in a community health center: A randomized, controlled trial. *Journal of General Internal Medicine* 24(2):211-217.

Roger, V. L., A. S. Go, D. M. Lloyd-Jones, R. J. Adams, J. D. Berry, T. M. Brown, M. R. Camethon, S. Dai, G. de Simone, E. S. Ford, C. S. Fox, H. J. Fullerton, C. Gillespie, K. J. Greenlund, S. M. Hailpem, J. A. Heit, P. M. Ho, V. J. Howard, B. M. Kissela, S. J. Kittner, D. T. Lackland, J. H. Lichtman, L. D. Lisabeth, D. M. Makuc, G. M. Marcus, A. Marelli, D. B. Matchar, M. M. McDermott, J. B. Meigs, C. S. Moy, D. Mozaffarian, M. E. Mussolino, G. Nichol, N. P. Paynter, W. D. Rosamond, P. D. Sorlie, R. S. Stafford, T. N. Turan, M. B. Turner, N. D. Wong, and J. Wylie-Rosett. 2011. Heart disease and stroke statistics—2011 update a report from the American Heart Association. *Circulation* 123(4):E18-E209.

Rohweder, C., M. Wolf, A. Schenck, V. Prasad, and S. Diehl. 2011. *Options for increasing colorectal cancer screening rates in North Carolina community health centers.* Chapel Hill, NC: UNC Lineberger Comprehensive Cancer Center.

U.S. Preventive Services Task Force. 2008. Screening for colorectal cancer: U.S. Preventive Services Task Force recommendation statement. *Annals of Internal Medicine* 149(9): 627-637.

Valery, L., O. Anke, K. K. Inge, and B. Johannes. 2008. Effectiveness of smoking cessation interventions among adults: A systematic review of reviews. *European Journal of Cancer Prevention* 17(6):535-544.

Yowell, A. 2011. Affordable Care Act Maternal, Infant, and Early Childhood Home Visiting Program. Presentation to the Committee on Integrating Primary Care and Public Health. Washington, DC.

# 4

# Policy and Funding Levers

Federal policy and funding are the greatest levers available to the Health Resources and Services Administration (HRSA) and the Centers for Disease Control and Prevention (CDC) to encourage the integration of primary care and public health on the ground. While the passage of the Patient Protection and Affordable Care Act (ACA) is arguably the most significant health policy event since the creation of Medicare and Medicaid in 1965, other advocacy and legislative efforts have recently been undertaken that create opportunities for primary care and public health to work together. These efforts attest to the momentum that exists for improving the health system, as well as the commitment to incorporating population health goals into health policy.

One of the policy efforts endorsed by the Obama administration is "place-based initiatives." As explained in a memorandum:

> Place-based policies leverage investments by focusing resources in targeted places and drawing on the compounding effect of well-coordinated action. Effective place-based policies can influence how rural and metropolitan areas develop, how well they function as places to live, work, operate a business, preserve heritage, and more. Such policies can also streamline otherwise redundant and disconnected programs. (The White House, 2009, p. 1)

The place-based initiatives policy is based on findings from social epidemiology that place-based factors act as determinants of health, independently of other factors (Poundstone et al., 2004). This policy recognizes that different approaches are needed for different geographic areas and that leveraging multiple actions with a shared goal has a cumulative effect. It also encourages agencies to cooperate in the development of initiatives and to coordinate funding streams. For example, the Sustainable Communities Regional Planning Grant Program is a collaborative effort of the Department of Housing and Urban Development, the Department of Transportation, and the Environmental Protection Agency to support planning for community improvement and address, among other issues, public and environmental health concerns.

Another effort under way is the Health in All Policies movement. Health in All Policies refers to the consideration of "health, well-being and equity during the development, implementation and evaluation of policies and services" (WHO, 2010, p. 2). It recognizes that policies that affect health often are not "health policies" per se; rather, policies in all sectors of society can affect the health of the population. For example, a study undertaken by the University of North Carolina (Bell and Standish, 2005) showed the positive impact on the dietary habits of surrounding African American communities when political and business decisions were made to relocate and facilitate access to supermarkets. The recent Institute of Medicine (IOM) report *For the Public's Health: Revitalizing Law and Policy to Meet New Challenges* (IOM, 2011b, p. 9) recommends that "states and the federal government develop and employ a Health In All Policies (HIAP) approach to consider the health effects—both positive and negative—of major legislation, regulations, and other policies that could potentially have a meaningful impact on the public's health."

Linked to the Health in All Policies concept is the health impact assessment, defined by the World Health Organization (WHO) as "a combination of procedures, methods, and tools by which a policy, program, or project may be judged as to its potential effects on the health of a population, and the distribution of those effects within the population" (European Centre for Health Policy, 1999, p. 4). Health impact assessments provide an assessment of the health effects of a policy prior to its implementation. Dannenberg and colleagues (2008) surveyed the use of health impact assessments in the United States and cited 27 examples, including one that examined the socioeconomic effects of an after-school program in Los Angeles; another that examined how a rental voucher program for low-income families in Massachusetts impacted housing affordability, housing stability, and the neighborhood environment; and another that looked at the effects of a community redevelopment project on physical activity. A recent report of the National Research Council (2011) describes the growing popularity of health impact assessments in the United States and proposes a framework for organizing and explaining their necessary elements.

An example of a legislative effort focused on health system improvement is the American Recovery and Reinvestment Act (ARRA) of 2009.

Designed as an economic stimulus bill, ARRA included approximately $150 billion directed at health and health care (Steinbrook, 2009). In addition to $87 billion for Medicaid and $1.1 billion for comparative effectiveness research, a few other programs are worth mentioning. For example, $2 billion was allocated to HRSA for health centers, specifically for construction, equipment, health information technology, and the provision of services; $1 billion was allocated for prevention and wellness, including clinical and community-based prevention activities designed to address chronic diseases; and the National Health Service Corps and other HRSA-supported workforce programs received $500 million.

Also included in ARRA was the Health Information Technology for Economic and Clinical Health (HITECH) Act, designed to improve the way the health care system operates (Blumenthal, 2010) by encouraging the collection and use of patient-level data through electronic health records. Using these data to inform population-level policies is one way in which primary care practices and public health departments can work together around a shared goal. Although many of ARRA's provisions ended after 2 years, it is important to recognize that even before the ACA became law, there was a movement to invest in and improve the nation's health system.

The remainder of this chapter examines provisions of the ACA, key policy components that should be incorporated into future legislation to facilitate the integration of primary care and public health, and funding streams that provide levers for achieving integration.

## THE PATIENT PROTECTION AND AFFORDABLE CARE ACT

That the ACA touches on virtually every aspect of health policy that has been debated over the last 25 years belies its expeditious and opportunistic origin. As a legislative feat, the ACA stands on its own merit. As an all-encompassing piece of health policy that addresses the potential to institutionalize population health, it is an incomplete blueprint.

In all fairness, the very title of the law speaks to its main aim—to safeguard health insurance coverage "for those that have it" and to make health insurance more affordable and accessible to the 51.5 million nonelderly Americans who are medically uninsured (Carrier et al., 2011). The majority of the act's provisions deal with health insurance reform and regulations and the structural basis for enabling those who have been crowded out of affordable health insurance to obtain coverage.

Within the building blocks of this reconstruction of Americans' health care coverage are policy elements covering the health care workforce and its training; innovation in care delivery; health disparities; data mining; and renewed investments in primary care, public health, and prevention. While these provisions were well promulgated, the ACA neither set out to nor provides a strategy to achieve population health improvement. Similarly, it does not explicitly address the integration of primary care and public health. Instead, it provides a menu of initiatives on which agencies and communities might converge to make gains in improving population health.

The ACA, by being about health insurance reform at its core, suggests that the long-term success of expanded insurance coverage must be accompanied by a set of activities that reset the basis on which health care is considered and rendered. In other words, health insurance deals only with payment of medical costs, whereas population health investments provide an opportunity for containing and maintaining health care costs within an affordable trajectory. The committee believes that within the numerous provisions of the ACA lie the seeds of opportunity to catalyze the integration of primary care and public health and embed population health improvement as an objective in achieving wellness and health for Americans.

Of particular note, the ACA authorizes both HRSA and CDC to launch a number of new programs that on their own merit promise to be noteworthy, but if coordinated and managed collaboratively from their inception could generate significant momentum toward population health improvement at the national, state, and local levels. In its review of HRSA and CDC activities in the ACA, the committee sought to identify provisions with the potential to yield long-lasting change in the integration of primary care and public health. Although other Department of Health and Human Services (HHS) agencies, notably the Centers for Medicare & Medicaid Services (CMS), and other federal departments and agencies have significant roles to play in promulgating a population health perspective, HRSA and CDC have unique roles under health care reform.

Ultimately, the extent to which HRSA and CDC are able to build upon this movement toward population health improvement is as much dependent on how these agencies, and more generally HHS, operate as on how they implement new programs. Leadership in the two agencies will need to reinvent the process and culture for implementing categorical grant programs, meeting congressional mandates, and complying with regulations while spurring the collaboration and cross-cutting accountability that are critical to establishing population health improvement as an operational imperative.

The following subsections highlight what the committee believes are particularly promising opportunities within the ACA. They fall into four categories: community investments and benefits, coverage reforms, health care transformation, and reshaping of the workforce.

## Community Investments and Benefits

The ACA makes direct investments in community health transformation and brings new focus to community benefit activities.

### Community Transformation Grants

The Community Transformation Grants program,[1] established through allocations from the Prevention and Public Health Fund, is a particularly compelling example of a public health-led initiative that could be used to integrate primary care and public health. The program consists of two parts: Community Transformation Grants and a National Network.

Community Transformation Grants have been awarded to 61 state and local government agencies, tribes and territories, and national and community-based organizations (CDC, 2011). The goal of the program is to reduce chronic disease rates, prevent secondary conditions, reduce health disparities, and assist in developing a stronger evidence base for effective prevention programs. These goals are to be met by supporting the implementation, evaluation, and dissemination of community preventive health activities that are grounded in evidence. Implemented by CDC, the program will support up to 75 communities across the country over a 5-year period, with projects increasingly expanding their scope and reach if federal resources allow. Funding is available for capacity building or implementation, and activities must grow out of an area health assessment (HHS, 2011).

Under CDC guidelines, the Community Transformation Grants program gives priority to the prevention and reduction of type 2 diabetes and the control of high blood pressure and cholesterol. Clinical preventive services are embedded in the basic structure of the Community Transformation Grants program, making health care providers a core partner in the types of broad-based coalitions whose involvement is essential to the program. All applicants are expected to focus on tobacco-free living; active living and healthy eating; and increased use of high-impact, quality clinical preventive services. Applicants also may choose to address social and emotional wellness and a healthy and safe physical environment (HHS, 2011).

The National Network is aimed at community-based organizations that are positioned to accelerate the speed with which communities adopt promising approaches to health transformation. Under the award program, network members can carry out this dissemination activity in two ways: first, by disseminating Community Transformation Grants strategies to their partners and affiliates, and second, by supporting and funding sub-

---

[1]*Patient Protection and Affordable Care Act of 2010 (ACA)*, Public Law 148, 111th Cong., 2d sess. § 4201 (March 23, 2010).

recipients in the use of Community Transformation Grants strategies to initiate change locally. Support for subrecipients can include helping them create leadership teams and providing technical assistance and guidance.

The Community Transformation Grants program and the National Network share a set of important purposes: to launch multiple interventions whose goal is making fundamental improvements in population health; to lessen the burden on the health care system while achieving its central involvement in the effort; to develop a new approach to the collection and use of public health information in order to bring an immediacy and action orientation to long-standing surveillance practices; and to accelerate the rate at which public health innovations are replicated nationally, regardless of whether the replication sites receive support from the Community Transformation Grants program. In this sense, the Community Transformation Grants program can be viewed as the public health counterpart to the CMS Innovation Center (CMMI) discussed later in this chapter, whose mission is to test and speed the acceleration of health care system transformation. Nowhere in the ACA is this potential parallelism developed more deeply, and it would be advantageous for both HRSA and CDC to be aware of the communities in which the Community Transformation Grants program and CMMI are involved. As community resources for wellness improve through the Community Transformation Grants program, it may be possible to begin to link those resources to CMMI pilots, which must be able to link their patients and physician practices to community resources. Similarly, the Community Transformation Grants sites will be important to HRSA in guiding health centers engaged in efforts to strengthen their clinical preventive service activities, including the development of affiliations with other community resources in such areas as nutrition, exercise, mental health and wellness, and cessation of tobacco use.

### Community Health Needs Assessments

One of the most important potential sources of community support created by the ACA may be the community benefit obligations of nonprofit hospitals that seek federal tax exempt status. A critical step HRSA and CDC might take jointly is a national collaboration with hospitals in ensuring that primary care and community health are given priority as hospitals move forward with their mandatory community health needs assessments and development of implementation strategies. Internal Revenue Service (IRS) guidelines in advance of formal regulations were issued in July 2011,[2] and the first mandatory reporting period for hospitals will be in 2012.

---

[2]IRS Notice 2011-52 (July 7, 2011).

In brief, section 501(c)(3) of the Internal Revenue Code[3] establishes the legal standard for determining whether nonprofit hospitals will be treated as tax exempt for federal income tax purposes. In 1969 the IRS issued Revenue Ruling 69-545,[4] which significantly rolled back previous reduced-cost care obligations in favor of a broader community benefit standard. This standard effectively went unenforced for years. In recent years, congressional scrutiny increased, culminating in amendments to the ACA[5] spelling out new obligations of all hospitals seeking federal tax exempt status (it is important to know that most state tax codes parallel the federal code). A 2006 Congressional Budget Office (CBO) report valued the total tax exemption at $12.6 billion in 2002 (CBO, 2006).

The ACA amends the Internal Revenue Code by adding new section 501(r), "additional requirements for certain hospitals."[6] The new requirements apply to all facilities licensed as hospitals, as well as organizations recognized by the Treasury Secretary as hospitals.[7] In the case of multihospital chains, each separate facility is held independently to the new requirements.[8] Hospitals failing to meet their obligations are subject to an excise tax of $50,000 for any taxable year in which they are not in compliance;[9] in addition, they will experience the adverse publicity of being found out of compliance.

The amendments impose new standards designed to ensure financial assistance to indigent persons, curb excessive charges for medically indigent patients, bar aggressive collection tactics, and ensure compliance with federal emergency care requirements. Of greatest interest to the committee is the obligation to undertake a community health needs assessment.

The community health needs assessment is a triennial process[10] that must commence no later than the taxable year 2 years after the ACA's enactment. The assessment must be accompanied by an implementation strategy that grows out of the needs assessment and, as discussed below, ongoing reporting on implementation efforts. The process is dynamic, evolving, and action oriented.

The ACA also establishes minimum requirements for the assessment itself. Under the law, an assessment must "take into account input from

---

[3]26 USC 501(c)(3).

[4]Rev. Rul. 69-545, 1969-2 C.B. 117. In the IRS's words, Revenue Ruling 69-545 "remove[d] the requirements relating to caring for patients without charge or at rates below cost" (Rev. Rul. 69-5454, 1969-2 C.B. 117).

[5]ACA § 9007 adding IRC § 501(r).

[6]ACA § 9007 adding IRC § 501(r), 26 U.S.C. § 501(r).

[7]Internal Revenue Code (IRC) § 501(r)(2).

[8]IRC § 501(r)(2)(C).

[9]IRC § 4959, added by ACA § 9007.

[10]IRC § 501(r)(3).

persons who represent the broad interests of the community served by the hospital facility" (IRS, 2011, p. 7). It is important to stress that the term used is "community," not the specific patients served by the hospitals. That is, the statute appears to require that hospitals assess the needs of the entire community covered by their service area, including members of the community who may, for a variety of reasons, receive care elsewhere, or receive no care at all. Furthermore, for a specialty hospital with a large geographic reach (e.g., a children's hospital or a hospital with a regional shock trauma unit), the needs assessment presumably will need to cover a community that is coextensive with this larger service area.

The development of the community health needs assessment must include individuals with public health expertise, thereby underscoring the obligation of facilities to involve knowledgeable individuals, not merely use public health data. In other words, the law emphasizes an assessment process that, with respect to both content and process, is inclusive of public health practice and expertise. Even the term "community health needs assessment" is drawn from the public health literature (see, e.g., Jordan et al., 1998; Robinson and Elkan, 1996), furthering the connection between hospital obligations and public health practice. While the legislative history refers to hospitals' ability to use public health information (Rosenbaum and Margulies, 2010), the text itself underscores the inclusive nature of the obligations.

The IRS's July 2011 notice reinforces these obligations, defining ambiguous terms and calling for an active and inclusive needs assessment process and, more important, an implementation strategy that is responsive to the needs assessment. The results of a needs assessment certainly could be reinvestment of hospital resources in uncompensated inpatient care discounts. But this would be the case only if the needs assessment were not carried out with heightened attention to primary care and community prevention needs. Hospitals now have a reason to focus on these investments as well, given the emergence of a Medicare payment policy that penalizes excessive readmissions and that serves as a model for state Medicaid programs and private payers. Accordingly, it may be possible for HRSA and CDC to engage with community hospitals and national hospital associations in developing approaches to hospital community benefit planning and implementation strategies that can support the types of activities touched on in this report for which sufficient investment funding is lacking. Examples of these activities include the extension of primary care services into nontraditional settings; the formation of collaboratives among community primary care providers and local health departments, with the aim of strengthening primary care; community health promotion activities involving diet, exercise, and injury risk reduction; and other population-level interventions.

## Coverage Reforms

When the ACA is fully implemented, it will expand coverage under Medicaid and the Children's Health Insurance Program (CHIP) to 17 million Americans and reduce the number of uninsured to 23 million (CBO, 2011). Americans with incomes below 133 percent of the poverty level will be eligible for Medicaid coverage (CBO, 2011; The Henry J. Kaiser Family Foundation, 2011).

### Medicaid Preventive Services

One of the ACA's provisions concerns preventive services for Medicaid populations. The ACA effectively creates two groups of eligible beneficiaries: individuals entitled to coverage under pre-ACA state plan standards and those entitled to coverage under the Medicaid eligibility expansion. In the case of traditional beneficiaries, the act clarifies that full coverage of all preventive services specified for privately insured persons is a state option and further incentivizes coverage through an increase in the federal medical assistance rate.[11] In the case of newly eligible adults, preventive services, as defined under the law, are a required element of Medicaid "benchmark" coverage, a somewhat different coverage standard from that used for the traditional population.[12]

In meeting this provision, primary care providers and public health departments can become participating Medicaid providers and furnish preventive services to adult and child populations. In addition, HRSA and CDC might consider collaborating with CMS on the development of joint guidance regarding coverage of preventive services. Such guidance might explain both the required and optional preventive service provisions of the law, as well as federal financing incentives for coverage of such services. The guidance also might describe best practices in making preventive services more accessible to Medicaid beneficiaries through the use of expanded managed care provider networks; out-of-network coverage[13] in nontraditional locations such as schools, public housing, workplace sites, and other places; qualification criteria for participating providers; recruitment of providers; measurement of quality performance; and assessment of impact on population health.

The ACA establishes a grant program under which the secretary of HHS will award grants to states that seek to incentivize the use of preven-

---

[11]42 U.S.C. § 1396d(a)(13) and 1396d(b) as amended by ACA § 4106.

[12]42 U.S.C. § 1396u-7(b), as amended by ACA § 2001.

[13]Medicaid agencies are free under federal law to add out-of-network coverage for services also covered on an in-network basis. Many agencies take such an approach for certain types of services, such as school health services.

tive services by Medicaid beneficiaries.[14] The aim of the program is not simply increased participation in prevention programs but actual outcomes showing reduced health risks; thus, its purpose is to achieve behavioral change and scalability in other states. Program priorities include smoking cessation, weight loss, lower cholesterol and blood pressure, and avoidance of the onset of diabetes. Because of the serious shortage of Medicaid providers in many communities, HRSA and CDC have a crucial role to play in the implementation of state demonstrations, particularly in outreach to community providers, training and technical support to state Medicaid agencies, active outreach to public health departments and health centers in demonstration states, and collaboration with CMS in the development of outcome standards and scalability criteria.

## Community Health Centers

One major challenge to the rapid expansion of health insurance coverage is the need for expanded capacity for primary care delivery (Adashi et al., 2010). In Massachusetts between 2005 and 2009, the number of uninsured individuals dropped from 657,000 to 295,000, and health centers and other safety net providers proved to be valuable assets in meeting the increased demand. Health centers' service volume increased by 31 percent. The uninsured in these practices fell from 35 percent to 19 percent, but by 2009, health centers were seeing 38 percent of all the uninsured in the state—up from 22 percent in 2005 (Ku et al., 2011).

The ACA and its companion Health Care and Education Reconciliation Act allocate a major infusion of funding to the expansion of health centers.[15] This is unquestionably one of the most important opportunities in the ACA to better integrate primary care and public health because of the unique practice characteristics of health centers. The original vision of health centers reflected what later came to be known as community-oriented primary care, that is, an approach to primary care practice that embeds public health principles into daily practice. These principles include needs assessments, prioritization of services based on population health characteristics, comprehensiveness, financial and cultural accessibility, evidence-based practice using tools such as modern health risk assessment approaches, continuous interaction with the community, and measurement of performance against community health goals, in addition to measures of individual patient-oriented clinical quality indicators. These aspirations still can be seen in the overall direction and management of health centers, but

---

[14]ACA § 4108.
[15]ACA § 5601.

health centers also have been under increasing pressure to improve clinical productivity, particularly in an era of limited resources.

An imperative for HRSA and CDC is to preserve the hybrid qualities of health centers and promote activities and linkages that maintain the health centers' primary role in clinical preventive services and community engagement. When possible, for example, health centers should be partners in Community Transformation Grants. Similarly, research on the experiences of health centers in the delivery of clinical preventive services is essential to understanding how the delivery of clinical preventive services might be improved for at-risk populations. Of necessity, outreach campaigns to promote clinical preventive services in underserved communities, as well as initiatives aimed at improving the quality of primary care for populations with serious and chronic health conditions, must focus on how to improve the performance of health centers.

Most important perhaps, every effort should be made to forge what often has been an uneasy relationship between health centers and public health departments. Many factors feed into this unease, including the historical roots of health centers as a counter to the segregation in health care that once pervaded a large region of the United States (Geiger, 2002, 2005), the fact that health centers have no direct legal financial accountability to health departments, and the different cultures found in health centers and public health departments. That said, there are instances in which partnerships between health centers and public health departments line up well. Typically, these are situations in which health departments have a declared interest in monitoring and intervening in the clinical care of patients who represent a perceived public health risk. For example, patients who are infected with tuberculosis (TB) can be managed by a primary care physician, but often public health departments are responsible for following up with patient contacts to establish the risk of spread in a given community. The level of public health intervention is likely to be even more pronounced if the patient is immunocompromised, as in the case of HIV-infected individuals, or if the patient has a case of active TB, with a high risk of infecting members of a community. In communities where TB is a significant public health concern, there can be explicit agreements between health centers and health departments regarding mutual notification of TB cases, care coordination, and follow-up. Similar arrangements may be in place for communities with high rates of sexually transmitted diseases.

In addition to areas that have traditionally provided opportunities for working together, such as infectious diseases and emergency preparedness, there are many anecdotal examples of collaboration between health centers and public health departments addressing the broader determinants of health. In California, for example, through the Black Infant Health Program, many health centers and public health departments worked to address high rates of infant mortality, particularly among African Americans (California Department of Public Health, 2010). Health centers, as a principal provider of prenatal care, work with public health departments to identify patients at risk. Maternal and child health workers are then deployed to provide home visits, make referrals to social service agencies, and promote maternal access to regular prenatal care. Such examples should be systematically identified; examined to determine their key elements; and replicated through collaborative efforts, much like the health disparities collaboratives developed by HRSA a decade ago. The failure of health centers and public health departments to act collaboratively would cost HRSA and CDC one of the greatest local levers for community change because their interests in population health are so aligned.

## Health Care Transformation

The ACA contains provisions whose aim is to stimulate new approaches to the organization and operation of health systems in order to improve effectiveness, efficiency, and quality.

### The National Prevention, Health Promotion and Public Health Council and the National Prevention Strategy

The National Prevention, Health Promotion and Public Health Council[16] provides coordination and leadership at the federal level to address health and efforts centered on disease prevention, wellness promotion, and public health. The council incorporates a broad view of health and accordingly comprises 17 different federal agencies, including HHS; the Departments of Agriculture, Education, Transportation, Labor, and Homeland Security; the Environmental Protection Agency; and others. The council is chaired by the Surgeon General. Its mission is to create a national strategy that identifies attainable goals for improving the health status of Americans and provides clear measures that will help agencies achieve those goals. Released in June 2011, the *National Prevention Strategy: America's Plan for Better Health and Wellness* (National Prevention, Health Promotion and Public Heath Council, 2011) promotes collaboration between stakeholders, and includes recommendations on the foundational elements of health (strategic directions) and on specific areas that strongly influence personal and public health (priorities). These strategic directions and priorities are listed in Box 4-1.

The National Prevention, Health Promotion and Public Health Council represents a mechanism through which HRSA and CDC can develop col-

---

[16]ACA § 4001.

---

**BOX 4-1**
**Strategic Directions and Priorities of the**
**National Prevention Strategy**

**Strategic Directions**

- Healthy and safe community environments
- Clinical and community preventive services
- Empowered people
- Elimination of health disparities

**Priorities**

- Tobacco-free living
- Preventing drug abuse and excessive alcohol use
- Healthy eating
- Active living
- Injury- and violence-free living
- Reproductive and sexual health
- Mental and emotional well-being

SOURCE: National Prevention, Health Promotion and Public Health Council, 2011.

---

laborations with each other and other federal agencies to impact the nation's health. As stated in the *National Prevention Strategy*, "the Council helps each agency incorporate health considerations into decision making, enhances collaboration on implementing prevention and health promotion initiatives, facilitates sharing of best practices, and, as appropriate, coordinates guidance and funding streams" (National Prevention, Health Promotion and Public Health Council, 2011, p. 8). By maximizing the potential of the council, HRSA and CDC could mount powerful initiatives, especially around the seven priorities. With the help of the Departments of Agriculture and Education, for example, CDC could aggressively target the implementation of healthier lunch options in schools. Likewise, HRSA could work with the Department of Transportation to fund programs that would provide transportation assistance to new mothers.

## CMS Innovation Center

The mission of CMMI[17] is to test new payment and service delivery models that advance clinical integration, health care quality, and efficiency. CMMI is intensely Medicare focused and therefore closely linked to the delivery of personal health care services. However, a number of community- and population-oriented approaches are being explored, indicating the potential for primary care and public health interaction. One of CMMI's enumerated areas of focus is "community and population health

---

[17]ACA § 3021.

models" (Center for Medicare and Medicaid Innovation, 2011). Through these models, CMMI can evaluate methods for linking the role of primary care to activities traditionally within the domain of public health, such as population-level behavioral interventions and prevention activities. To the extent that this has not already occurred, HRSA and CDC could engage with CMMI in the identification of community and population health models. In the provisions of the law that focus on CMMI and elsewhere in the ACA, a major thrust of health care reform is attention to dually eligible Medicare and Medicaid beneficiaries. The population dually eligible for these programs has been a special concern for CMS and, to a lesser extent, CMMI, state Medicaid programs, the Medicaid and CHIP Payment and Access Commission (MACPAC), the Medicare Payment Advisory Commission (MedPAC), and Congress. HRSA and CDC could target these dually eligible beneficiaries by developing an initiative aimed at improving their health and health care. In HRSA's case, health centers represent one of the most important sources of care for these populations, while CDC's expertise in chronic disease measurement is important as well. Local health departments may have a central role to play in creating the types of practice support environments and tools that are essential to transforming the quality of care available to dual enrollees.

*Accountable Care Organizations*

The ACA establishes accountable care organizations (ACOs) as a formally defined approach to health care practice as part of the new Medicare Shared Savings Program.[18] The ACO model grew out of recommendations by MedPAC (MedPAC, 2009) aimed at introducing practice management techniques that can increase health care quality and efficiency while achieving improved health outcomes across a broad patient population. CMS's final rule, issued in fall 2011 (CMS, 2011), was revised significantly in response to voluminous comments on the administration's initial approach to implementation, which included allowing federally qualified health centers (FQHCs) and rural health clinics to participate in ACOs, as well as form independent ACOs. The final rule stipulates that ACOs that meet quality and savings goals can keep a percentage of the savings. This provision is designed to encourage participating providers to redesign their practices innovatively and include a focus on improved health for populations (U.S. National Archives and Records Administration, 2011).

This provision creates the opportunity for a partnership between HRSA and CDC around safety net ACOs and public health departments. HRSA might encourage health centers to create their own ACOs or align with

---

[18]Social Security Act § 1899, added by ACA § 3022.

other ACOs that may be forming in their communities and support collaboration with health departments in these institutions. To the extent that health centers move in this direction, HRSA and CDC might develop collaboration models between health centers acting as and collaborating with other ACOs and public health departments. Such collaboration models might emphasize the role of public health in needs assessment, performance measurement and improvement, health promotion, and patient engagement, all of which are central elements of ACOs.

## Patient-Centered Medical Homes and the Community Health Team

Patient-centered medical homes are defined in Section 3502 of the ACA as a mode of care that includes "(a) personal physicians or other primary care providers; (b) whole person orientation; (c) coordinated and integrated care; (d) safe and high-quality care through evidence-informed medicine, appropriate use of health information technology, and continuous quality improvements; (e) expanded access to care; and (f) payment that recognizes added value from additional components of patient-centered care."[19] These "homes" are designed to care for the whole person as a complex system of needs and challenges and provide a continuum of care that encourages healthy living and a healthy lifestyle. Patient-centered medical homes are supported by "community health teams," a concept that is established and supported by grant funding under the ACA. Section 3502 also authorizes the secretary of HHS to award community health team grants or contracts to eligible entities for the establishment of community-based interdisciplinary, interprofessional teams (health teams), which support primary care providers and receive capitated payments for their services. The model is based on prior work by health care experts who have focused on the task of strengthening the capacity of the primary health care system to address the highest-cost patients (IOM, 2010; Wagner, 2000). This strengthening of capacity is envisioned as not simply upgrading practice but essentially embedding practice in a broader public health model. Entities eligible for grants are state or tribal entities that can demonstrate a plan for long-term financial sustainability and a plan for incorporating prevention initiatives, patient education, and care management resources into the delivery of health care in a highly integrated fashion.[20] Teams must be interdisciplinary; the statute contains references to the full range of medical, nursing, nutritional, social work, and mental health professionals. Most important, teams must agree to serve not only Medicare beneficiaries but also Medicaid beneficiaries receiving care through state medical home initiatives.

---

[19]ACA § 3502.
[20]ACA § 3502.

Numerous challenges arise, all of which create collaboration opportunities for HRSA and CDC working with state and local health departments, health centers, and professional organizations. These challenges involve creating the teams; developing team practice approaches that fulfill all requirements of the law with respect to team composition and the scope, depth, and range of activities, community support services, and performance reporting; and integrating public health and public health work into the team model. Primary care providers must be enlisted, collaborations must be developed, health information technology must be utilized, and practice performance must be measured. The most significant challenge may be developing sustainability models for Medicare and Medicaid that can be translated into private health insurance and across varying population demographics. At the same time, the potential to transform community primary care practice into a model that can better manage the highest-risk populations through partnerships between private professionals and public health departments and safety net providers is great.

### Reshaping of the Workforce

In the context of system transformation, the ACA falls short in the area of workforce improvement. Yet while major workforce investments are absent in the law, there are some opportunities for reshaping the workforce that HRSA and CDC, working together, could exploit.

#### Primary Care Extension Program

The ACA authorizes the Agency for Healthcare Research and Quality (AHRQ) to establish the Primary Care Extension Program (PCEP). This program is modeled after the U.S. Department of Agriculture's Cooperative Extension Program, which revolutionized farming over the last decade, speeding the translation of research to plow and bringing learning from innovative farms back to universities (Grumbach and Mold, 2009; Vastag, 2004). The PCEP can help speed the transformation of care based on best evidence, whether from research or from innovative practices. PCEP agents will establish relationships with practices, much as pharmaceutical representatives did during the last 50 years, but with a detailing function geared to incorporating evidence-based techniques, preventive medicine, health promotion, chronic disease management, and mental and behavioral health services into primary care practices. The goal is to facilitate adoption of the principles of the patient-centered medical home and population health management. AHRQ funded four existing state-based PCEP programs, three of which are required to help three additional states develop similar PCEP programs (the fourth also needs to be scalable to other states). Thus, more than 13 states will be involved in PCEP efforts over the next 2 years (AHRQ, 2010). Fully fledged, the PCEP could function through grants received by PCEP State Hubs and Local Primary Care Extension Agencies. The State Hubs could include state health departments, state Medicaid and Medicare program administrators, and the departments of academic institutions that train providers in primary care. In addition to these entities, State Hubs might include such entities as hospital associations, primary care practice-based research networks, and state primary care associations. Local Primary Care Extension Agencies are required to perform a number of tasks under the ACA. These tasks include assisting primary care providers in implementing the principles of the patient-centered medical home model, developing and supporting primary care learning communities to enhance dissemination of best practices and improve the involvement of local providers in research, and developing a plan for financial sustainability after the scheduled reduction of federal funding.

While the PCEP is the domain of AHRQ, HRSA and CDC have many reasons to work with AHRQ to elevate the PCEP to a priority within HHS and seek collaboration with CMMI to fund PCEP models that evidence shows can improve personal and population health. The ACA expressly mentions that the PCEP could help support health centers, rural health clinics, and National Health Service Corps (NHSC) sites. In addition, the PCEP could be a bridge between primary care and public health in every county of the country. Once more mature, the PCEP could "participate in community-based efforts to address the social and broad determinants of health, strengthen the local primary care workforce, and eliminate health disparities."[21] In working with AHRQ, HRSA and CDC could help ensure that the program includes a public health orientation and integrates community health issues into practice- and clinic-based primary care improvement activities. For these mutual reasons, the three agencies could build a case for why HHS should support the program, and could also provide guidance on the development of measures for evaluating the program's effectiveness in involving public health in clinical practice.

## National Health Service Corps

The NHSC,[22] whose loan and scholarship recipients constitute a significant proportion of all health professionals in health center practice, has received an important infusion of funding. Given the goals of clinical preventive services, one important area of collaboration between HRSA and CDC might be in prioritizing the recruitment and placement of NHSC

---

[21]ACA § 5405. p. 584.
[22]ACA § 5207.

resources. NHSC loan and scholarship recipients play a vital role in the staffing of health centers. To the extent that other practice sites are feasible, combining information on designated health professions shortage areas with community public health data on community-wide health risks could guide the selection of placement sites. HRSA and CDC may want to explore linkages between the NHSC and the Epidemic Intelligence Service (EIS), particularly with EIS officers placed in state and local health departments (the EIS is discussed further later in the chapter).

*Teaching Health Centers*

Although virtually all workforce development provisions of the ACA face the prospect of no implementation funding, one provision that did receive an appropriation under the act is the teaching health centers program.[23] A teaching health center is defined as a community-based patient care center that operates a residency program. Teaching health centers expand training in FQHCs and rural health clinics to expose resident physicians to caring for the underserved. The training expansion grants include physicians ($167.3 million), physician assistants ($30.1 million), and advanced practice nurses ($31 million). The program is limited to 5 years of funding and then will expire (HHS, 2010).

Because entities must operate a residency training program to qualify for developmental grants and the special payment programs, the focus of the award itself is on training programs that can demonstrate a strong community basis—formal affiliations and partnerships with entities such as health centers, urban Indian health clinics, and other community health care providers that have strong community roots and can share in the direction and oversight of the program. The teaching health centers program not only awards grants for the development of centers but, more important, provides ongoing training support through a mandatory appropriation that is part of the ACA.

Collaboration between HRSA and CDC might merit particular attention in examining the possibilities for teaching health centers. For example, all teaching health centers might be linked to community transformation activities in communities that receive Community Transformation Grants, discussed earlier. Centers also could benefit from the national educational component of the Community Transformation Grants program in order to learn about models of integration that are working and could be replicated in other communities.

Teaching health centers presumably would be ideal locations for en-

---

[23]ACA § 5508, *Public Health Act of 1944*, Public Law 410, 78th Cong. 2d sess. § 749A (July 1, 1944).

suring access to the clinical preventive services that must be part of all programs funded by Community Transformation Grants. HRSA and CDC might consider working with the centers on training programs whose aim is to produce competency to work in community health teams, given the emphasis placed on teams under the ACA. Teaching health center programs and residents also might focus on health care for dual enrollees, given the large number of health center sites that undoubtedly will serve high concentrations of low-income Medicare beneficiaries.

In sum, the teaching health centers program offers HRSA and CDC an opportunity to address the shortage of providers trained in a model of primary care that incorporates principles of public health practice and emphasizes the management of populations that are the most difficult to serve and whose clinical challenges may be matched only by their social needs. Exploiting this opportunity may be particularly important given that the funding to support the residency placements is set to expire.

While by no means a complete list of relevant provisions in the ACA, Table 4-1 presents an overview of those provisions the committee believes offer the most promising opportunities for HRSA and CDC to work together to foster the integration of primary care and public health.

**TABLE 4-1** Selected Provisions of the Patient Protection and Affordable Care Act That Offer Opportunities for HRSA and CDC

| Affordable Care Act Provision | HRSA and CDC Opportunities |
| --- | --- |
| Community Transformation Grants (ACA §§ 4002 and 4201) The provision authorizes and funds community transformation grants to improve community health activities and outcomes. | • Given that Community Transformation Grants can be viewed as the public health counterpart to the Centers for Medicare & Medicaid Services (CMS) Innovation Center (CMMI) pilots, HRSA and CDC should be aware of the communities where both of these programs are involved.<br>• As community resources for wellness improve through the Transformation Grant system, it may be possible to encourage state and local health department recipients to develop linkages with primary care providers as a central focus of their program planning.<br>• CDC could also begin to link those resources to CMMI pilots, which must be able to link their patients and physician practices with community resources. |

*continued*

**TABLE 4-1** Continued

| Affordable Care Act Provision | HRSA and CDC Opportunities |
| --- | --- |
| Community Health Needs Assessments (ACA § 9007) The provision amends the Internal Revenue Code by adding new section 501(r), "additional requirements for certain hospitals." The new requirements apply to all facilities licensed as hospitals and organizations recognized by the Treasury secretary as hospitals and spell out new obligations for all hospitals seeking federal tax exempt status. | • HRSA and CDC could engage with community hospitals and national hospital associations to develop approaches to hospital community benefit planning, as well as promote approaching jointly the selection of interventions and implementation strategies to address identified problems—for example, the extension of primary care services into nontraditional settings; the formation of collaboratives among community primary care providers and local public health and other agencies; and community health promotion activities involving diet, exercise, and injury risk reduction, as well as other population-level interventions. |
| Medicaid Preventive Services (ACA §§ 4106 and 2001) (ACA § 4108) The provision gives states the option to improve coverage of clinical preventive services for traditional eligibility groups, as well as Medicaid benchmark coverage for newly eligible persons, redefined to parallel the act's definition of essential health benefits, which includes coverage for preventive services. It also provides Medicaid incentives for prevention of chronic diseases. | • Primary care providers and public health departments could become participating Medicaid providers and collaborate in designing programs to furnish preventive services to adult and child populations.<br>• HRSA and CDC could collaborate with CMS on the development of joint guidance regarding coverage of preventive services. Such guidance might explain both the required and optional preventive service provisions of the law, as well as federal financing incentives for coverage of those services. Such guidance also might describe best practices in making preventive services more accessible to Medicaid beneficiaries through the use of expanded managed care provider networks and out-of-network coverage in nontraditional locations such as schools, public housing, and workplace sites; qualification criteria for participating providers; recruitment of providers; measurement of quality performance; and assessment of impact on population health.<br>• HRSA and CDC have a crucial role to play in the implementation of state demonstrations, particularly in outreach to community providers to enlist them as active participants in such demonstrations, training and technical support to state Medicaid agencies, outreach to public health departments and health centers in demonstration states, and collaboration with CMS on the development of outcome standards and scalability criteria. |

**TABLE 4-1** Continued

| Affordable Care Act Provision | HRSA and CDC Opportunities |
| --- | --- |
| Community Health Centers (ACA § 5601) The provision expands funding for health centers. | • An imperative for HRSA is to preserve and strengthen the role of health centers as core safety net providers of clinical care and prevention in the communities they serve. Incentives could be built into funding for these centers to promote activities and linkages with local public health departments and encourage community engagement and partnerships for community-based prevention. <br> • Outreach campaigns to promote clinical preventive services in underserved communities, as well as initiatives aimed at improving the quality of primary care for populations with serious and chronic health conditions, could focus on how to improve the performance of health centers. |
| National Prevention, Health Promotion and Public Health Council and the National Prevention Strategy (ACA § 4001) The provision creates the National Prevention, Health Promotion and Public Health Council to create a collaborative national strategy to address health in the nation. | • HRSA and CDC could use the Council as a mechanism for working with other agencies around the integration of primary care and public health. |
| CMS Innovation Center (CMMI) (ACA § 3021) The provision establishes CMMI to develop, conduct, and evaluate pilots for improving quality, efficiency, and patient health outcomes in both the Medicare and Medicaid programs, with an emphasis on dual enrollees. | • HRSA and CDC could engage with CMMI in the implementation of its community health innovation program to develop models that would leverage clinical care to achieve a broader impact on population health. <br> • In the CMMI provisions of the ACA and elsewhere in the act, a major thrust of health care reform is attention to dually eligible Medicare/Medicaid beneficiaries. HRSA and CDC could develop an initiative aimed at improving the health and health care of this population. |

*continued*

**TABLE 4-1** Continued

| Affordable Care Act Provision | HRSA and CDC Opportunities |
| --- | --- |
| Accountable Care Organizations (ACOs) (ACA § 3022) The provision authorizes the secretary of the Department of Health and Human Services (HHS) to enter into agreements with ACOs on a shared savings basis to improve the quality of patient care and health outcomes and increase efficiency. | • HRSA could encourage health centers to form ACOs and link with public health departments in this endeavor.<br>• HRSA and CDC could develop models of collaboration between public health departments and ACOs that include safety net providers. Such models might emphasize the role of public health in needs assessment, performance measurement and improvement, health promotion, and patient engagement, all of which are central elements of ACOs. |
| Patient-Centered Medical Homes (ACA § 3502) The provision authorizes state Medicaid programs to establish medical homes for Medicaid beneficiaries with chronic health conditions, and authorizes the secretary of HHS to award grants for the establishment of health teams to support primary care. | • HRSA and CDC could collaborate on further development of the medical home model and its team-based approach to care and encourage the inclusion of local public health departments in that model.<br>• HRSA and CDC could provide technical support to state Medicaid agencies seeking to pursue the medical home model, imparting best practices in the design and development of a medical home that is comprehensive, efficient in care delivery, and patient/family-centered. This support also could be expanded to include the development of performance measurement tools for measuring progress in these areas.<br>• HRSA and CDC could develop a sustainable model for the medical home in Medicare and Medicaid that encourages inclusion of local public health departments, supports multiple population types, and can be translated for private health insurance as well. |
| Primary Care Extension Program (ACA § 5405) The provision authorizes the Agency for Healthcare Research and Quality (AHRQ) to award competitive grants to states for the establishment of Primary Care Extension Programs to improve the delivery of primary care and community health. | • HRSA and CDC could work with AHRQ to ensure that Primary Care Extension Programs include a public health orientation and integrate community health issues into practice- and clinic-based primary care improvement activities.<br>• HRSA and CDC, working jointly with AHRQ, could seek collaboration with CMMI to fund Primary Care Extension Program models for which there is evidence for improving personal and population health. |

**TABLE 4-1** Continued

| Affordable Care Act Provision | HRSA and CDC Opportunities |
|---|---|
| National Health Service Corps (ACA § 5207) The provision expands funding for the National Health Service Corps. | • HRSA and CDC could collaborate in prioritizing the recruitment and placement of National Health Service Corps resources and developing linkages with existing Epidemic Intelligence Service (EIS) officers placed in state and local health departments. |
| Teaching Health Centers (ACA § 5508) The provision authorizes and funds the establishment of and ongoing operational support for teaching health centers, which must be community-based. | • HRSA could work with teaching health centers to adopt the patient-centered medical home curriculum and ensure that any curriculum used to train residents includes strong community and public health components—ideally with residents working on projects that concretely promote primary care-public health integration.<br>• HRSA and CDC could work with the centers on training programs that would be aimed at producing competency to work in community health teams, given the emphasis placed on teams under the ACA. |

NOTE: ACA = Patient Protection and Affordable Care Act.

## KEY POLICY COMPONENTS

While the ACA does present some opportunities that can be leveraged to integrate primary care and public health, this was, as noted earlier, not its purpose. This section describes key policy components that should be considered for incorporation into future legislation as a way to foster integration and begin to build an infrastructure that will facilitate the alignment of primary care and public health.

### Alignment of Payment and Incentive Structures to Encourage the Integration of Primary Care and Public Health

Creating momentum for the integration of primary care and public health will require changes in the way both are funded. Current primary care payment systems reward volume rather than value (Robert Wood Johnson Foundation et al., 2009). Fee-for-service payments create little incentive or accountability for individual patient outcomes, much less for monitoring and management of population health outcomes (Roland, 2004). Health care systems in the United States and in other countries that achieve better value in terms of quality and outcomes typically incentivize both measures of value through their payment systems (Roland, 2004). Most often, such payment systems include some form of capitation, frequently as a blend of fee-for-service and per-member-per-month payment and rewards for measurable reporting of care measures or actual outcomes. In systems or countries that outperform the United States broadly, the capitated or blended payments to primary care providers often represent a larger proportion of total health care spending than is the case in the overall U.S. health care system (Campbell et al., 2007). In these better-performing systems, the rewards or incentives are also sizable and can make up a significant proportion of total revenue. This revenue often translates into increased income, but also reflects increased investment in the capacity of practices to deliver higher-quality care and to focus on the total health of their patient panel (Gulliford et al., 2007).

Funding for public health comes from a mix of federal, state, and local funds. An analysis by the Trust for America's Health (2011) found wide variability in funding amounts for states and localities, with no overarching strategy for directing funds to address the most pressing health needs. Moreover, most funding for public health is in the form of categorical grants, allowing grantees little flexibility. To promote integration with primary care, funding streams for public health should be flexible enough to encourage grantees to try innovative approaches to improving population health by partnering with primary care. Currently, payment for primary care services and funding for public health services neither align nor facilitate partnering.

While it may appear out of scope or capacity for HRSA or CDC to focus on payment or quality incentives, the two agencies have both an internal and an external role to play. HRSA has supported quality improvement efforts for safety net programs under its purview, for example, and currently hosts voluntary quality improvement technical assistance and accreditation support (HRSA, 2009). In addition, the grants it oversees through Section 330 of the Public Health Service Act[24] could be used to promote population health goals in health centers. As a condition for receiving 330 funds, for example, health centers could be asked to demonstrate awareness of the 10 essential public health services (Box 1-2 in Chapter 1), as well as provide access to and coverage for all preventive health services recommended by the U.S. Preventive Services Task Force. Through the National Center for Health Statistics and its ties to public health departments, CDC has an important role in presenting health outcomes and disparities by community. These two capacities could help in identifying areas with poor outcomes and high disparities in the vicinity of primary care safety net services and public health departments, and in developing incentives and support programs, alone and with Medicare and Medicaid, with a focus on joint interventions and ultimately integration. Where poor outcomes and large disparities exist without primary care safety net services, public health de-

---

[24]42 U.S.C. § 254b.

partments, or both, HRSA and CDC could work with CMS to create incentives for providers to locate in these areas, with strong incentives to create linkages with regional public health entities. In addition, as a condition for receipt of certain funds for state health departments, CDC could ask that they demonstrate awareness of and establish a working relationship with all safety net providers in their state.

### Investments That Grow and Reengineer a Workforce That Can Deliver on Population Outcomes

Orienting the U.S. health system to facilitate the integration of primary care and public health will require the development of a workforce that is capable of transcending the traditional boundaries of the two sectors to foster a collaborative environment. Workforce training initiatives have the potential to teach health professionals about the valuable interactions between personal and population-based health services and encourage relationships across disciplines. Specific training initiatives could include emphasizing team-based training, population health management competencies, epidemiology, and community-based health policy training within profession-specific training; training professionals in the community in practices that model integration and team-based care; training health care specialists to collaborate more closely with patients' primary care and community care teams; and expanding specialization in community-based epidemiology, geospatial health care analysis, population health management, practice transformation and improvement, and community care integration. A number of funding and policy opportunities already in place could assist in the development of a workforce with the capacity to carry out the principles of integration; however, the purpose of those funding opportunities may require significant changes.

Both HRSA and CDC could contribute to the creation of this workforce through their existing workforce programs. Since passage of the ACA, HRSA has made important investments to expand primary care training in 11 teaching health centers (discussed earlier) (HRSA, 2011) and a 5-year, $228 million expansion of primary care workforce training (HHS, 2010). HRSA also has a long-term stake in medical and nursing workforce pipeline programs covered by Titles VII and VIII of the Public Health Service Act. Title VII funds a number of programs, including predoctoral, residency, and faculty development training grants, as well as physician assistant programs. Title VIII provides similar support for nursing training. The Title VII programs focus on supporting primary care education programs that promote interprofessional education, training to meet the needs of a diverse population, and increased diversity in the workforce (Reynolds, 2008). HRSA also supports the development of the public health workforce through public health traineeships, public health training centers, and preventive medicine residency programs. In addition to building linkages between these existing HRSA programs, HRSA should consider partnering with CDC around its workforce programs.

The largest of CDC's workforce programs is the EIS, a 2year post-graduate training program that provides service and on-the-job learning for health professionals interested in the practice of applied epidemiology (CDC, 2012). The program is modeled after a traditional medical residency program, where much of the education occurs through experiential learning. About 75 percent of EIS graduates remain in public health at CDC or in state or local health departments, and many become field leaders around the world (CDC, 2012). While the EIS program currently is focused heavily on infectious diseases, it has the potential to fill an important gap in what is needed to achieve the goal of improving population health. With expansion of its scope and size, the EIS could create a public health workforce that could serve as a bridge between primary care and public health in two key areas: (1) transformation of primary care practice toward the capacity to monitor and manage population health, and (2) public health informatics and the capacity to turn patient and population health data into information that clinicians and public health workers can use to improve health in their communities.

The first of these areas could support the Primary Care Extension Program by helping practices learn how to use information technology to become better personal and population health managers within their practices. This assistance would include demonstrating how the new population health data streams can support clinical decisions at the point of care, as well as teaching health coaches or other practice health care workers how to use the new data streams to better manage and monitor chronically ill patients and coordinate preventive care services. Creating new population health information technology systems will not prepare clinics for using them effectively. An expanded EIS workforce could continue to employ sophisticated physician and nursing EIS agents but also develop a master of public health (MPH) and informatics cadre trained in the use of population health information technology systems at the community level—fulfilling their function for the public health system—and able to train practices in the use of these systems as an outreach from and bridge to public health. Within the public health system, their relationships with practices would help them understand how to connect partnering practices to patients or communities in their service area that were experiencing disparities in health. They could also bring public health resources to bear in determining how to assess and engage failing communities in partnership with practices. Fulfilling these obligations would require additional, specialized training for EIS agents. However, the benefit of expanding the skill set of those participating in the EIS program is that it would create a bridge between primary care and public health by broadening an existing program.

Another opportunity for HRSA and CDC to play an important role in workforce development is through interdisciplinary primary care and public health training. One means to this end would be to provide leadership to CMS in the development of related regulations for funding of graduate medical education and nurse training. The education advisory committees staffed by HRSA could be instrumental in providing this guidance. Many of the needed new or expanded functions in public and community health may best fall within the purview of CDC, especially those focused on turning personal and public health data into information that can drive interventions and practice improvement. HRSA and CDC should collaborate in reviewing their workforce programs to determine how they could be deployed to promote the production of health care workers who are able to integrate primary care and public health for the betterment of population health.

## Support for Population-Level Data

With the right design, important information to guide clinical decision making, public health interventions, and the integration of the two could be at the fingertips of health care providers. The advent of electronic health records may be seminal in introducing a new era of alignment between primary care and public health. HRSA has invested heavily in supporting the adoption of electronic health records among health centers, which in their full implementation will capture data for up to 20 million patients. Many of these health centers already have the means to capture some population health metrics, and a fully developed health information infrastructure at health centers should be capable of capturing information about population characteristics, as well as care management patterns and trends. Of course, health centers are not alone in undertaking the implementation of electronic health records. Through a myriad of initiatives, including "meaningful use" incentives administered by the Office of the National Coordinator, the United States is being ushered into the digital era of health care. Whether the full potential of this enterprise in generating population health improvement will be realized remains to be seen. But undeniably, the elements of success are there: a desire to reinvest in new models of care delivery with primary care at its core; an understanding that health care costs will continue to escalate uncontrollably unless prevention and social determinants are addressed; and the technological means to capture information that can serve the dual goals of improved clinical care and optimized population health, as well as create a link between the two (although it should be noted that the investment in health information technology for public health has been significantly less than the investment for primary care) (Steinbrook, 2009).

In *For the Public's Health: The Role of Measurement in Action and Accountability* (IOM, 2011a, p. 2), the IOM states "that the United States lacks a coherent template for population health information that could be used to understand the health status of Americans and to assess how well the nation's efforts and investments result in improved population health." To gauge performance in addressing health disparities and improving population health, well-developed measures are needed at all levels—local, state, and national. Efforts to develop measures, coordinate data collection, analyze outcomes, and translate this information for decision makers are being undertaken in some locations. In the Geisinger system, optimal outcomes were identified and used as the basis for developing short- and long-term metrics. This approach, along with the use of real-time data from electronic health records and insurance claims, has contributed to improved outcomes and cost reductions (Steele et al., 2010). Another example is WellMed, a primary care-based ACO in Texas. The measurement and accountability systems WellMed has implemented have contributed to lowered mortality rates and better outcomes compared with state outcomes for the over-65 population (Phillips et al., 2011).

In contrast to these examples, in which coordination was crucial to success, efforts currently under way by CMS, the National Committee for Quality Assurance, certifying boards, and payers are disjointed. The efforts undertaken by the various stakeholders could be coordinated and structured to become a routine part of patient care.

In addition to coordination, an important element related to metrics is how the collected data are used. Ideally, measures should be used as a feedback loop in the provision of care, giving providers quality measures for their patient panel, and perhaps even as decision support at the point of care. Collected data also can be used to identify groups or communities with poor outcomes that may be small in number or distributed across multiple practices, and therefore not easily recognized by individual practices. Aggregated data can be used to identify these groups so they can be targeted by collaborative outreach, engagement, and improved services.

## Shared Community Resources for Primary Care and Public Health Integration

The most important way to encourage the integration of primary care and public health is to prevent further erosion of either sector. As states seek to reduce health care spending, public health funding is an easy target for program cuts. One way to combat these cuts is to physically unite or collocate public health departments with local health centers. Doing so would reduce the infrastructure costs of maintaining separate operating resources. Also, communities could find ways to join public health initiatives with primary care practices. For instance, HRSA could recommend the use of public health workers in health centers as community agents responsible for patient education, behavioral and lifestyle modification, and assistance to patient communities in overcoming social determinants that adversely affect community health. These workers could utilize training and tools developed by CDC to achieve these goals, and would be responsible for relaying community health metrics to CDC and state and local health departments for inclusion in local, state, and national data reports. These shared resources, embedded in the community and community relationships, would help provide complex care management; assist with practice transformation, health information technology connectivity, care, and coordination of community services; and assist in monitoring the health of the public. This consolidation also could provide an opportunity for patients to receive all of their personal care and public health services in one stop and lead to improved economies of scale due to shared space, shared resources, and shared staff.

Another opportunity for sharing community resources is around workforce. For example, the Vermont Blueprint for Health employs community care teams as a link between primary care practices and public health services, including community-based chronic disease prevention programs, as well as social and economic support programs. While team composition is determined locally, all teams are led by a nurse, and most consist of behavioral health counselors and social workers (Bielaszka-DuVernay, 2011). Community care teams can be based in primary care practices and assist patients with such tasks as making appointments, completing insurance paperwork, or arranging child care. Thus, these teams ensure that people have comprehensive services to support their health and well-being by connecting the work of primary care practices to community-based preventive and other social services.

Box 4-2 presents some examples in which sharing of community resources to support the integration of primary care and public health is working well.

The shared capacity to use patient and population data is another example of a resource available to promote the integration of primary care and public health. Important efforts are under way at HRSA to share patient data in a safe way (compliant with the Health Insurance Portability and Accountability Act [HIPAA]) and combine them with population data to produce information of value to practices and communities. While HRSA is making these efforts, CDC could work to ensure that its data analyses are not so far removed from the community level as to be of little use to providers at the local level. To this end, it may be necessary to develop programs that not only aggregate data to the state and national levels

---

**BOX 4-2**
**Examples of Shared Community Resources**

In Yavapai County, Arizona, Community Health Services oversees both the community health center and the public health department. Community Health Services promotes the integration of the two by collocating services in the same buildings and using their separate boards as a vehicle for bridging their activities. The County Board of Supervisors, the community health center board, and the board of health have overlapping representation, including the same physician, nurse, and county representative (Personal communication, Robert Resendes, Director of Yavapai County Community Health Services, March 28, 2011).

Hudson River HealthCare, a primary care network in upstate New York, uses an innovative workforce to link with public health. Patient care partners assist patients with prescription assistance programs, referrals to outside agencies, and food and Special Supplemental Nutrition Program for Women, Infants, and Children (WIC) assistance, as well as patient education and self-management support. Community care partners provide similar services but are physically located in the community. They work in homeless shelters, after-school programs, community centers, and hospital emergency rooms. Hudson River HealthCare considers staff working in both of these positions to be integral to its work (Personal communication, Kathy Brieger, CEO, Hudson River HealthCare, May 2, 2011).

---

but also are capable of disaggregating the data based on geographic location and patient composition, as well as a nationally accessible platform for storing and disseminating these data. This disaggregation, which could be done at the state and local levels, would allow primary care providers not only to view their geographic population, but also to compare their population with similar populations across the state and nation. Currently, most practices lack the fundamental capability to turn their patient data into information that allows them to compare their practice with the practices of peers, to identify learning opportunities and areas of shared concern, and to look at their data in the context of community. Shared data resources, particularly with an analytic component to keep the data sharing safe and useful, would be important for primary care and public health integration.

## FUNDING STREAMS

In addition to legislation, funding streams can be used as a lever to encourage integration. To better understand this lever, it is helpful to understand the role of HRSA and CDC (as well as CMS) in funding health centers and health departments.

## Funding for Health Centers and Health Departments

Health centers, state health departments, and local health departments receive revenue from a variety of sources. Figures 4-1, 4-2, and 4-3 show the average sources of revenue for health centers, state health departments, and local health departments, respectively. While the data do not reveal whether federal funding was primarily from HRSA or CDC, the nature of the two agencies' activities suggests the likely source: federal direct and pass-through funding for health centers would be supplied primarily by HRSA, while federal funding received by state and local health departments could be assumed to be received primarily from CDC.

Figure 4-1 shows that federal direct and pass-through funding accounted for only 23.2 percent of health center revenues in 2010[25] (Kaiser Family Foundation, 2010). The other 78 percent comprises Medicare and Medicaid funding (5.8 and 37.7 percent, respectively), other public and private insurance (9.5 percent), direct payment by users (5.9 percent), and other funds provided through state and local grants and contracts and other sources (Kaiser Family Foundation, 2010).

Figure 4-2 shows that in 2009, 45 percent of state health departments' budgets were derived from federal funding, with an additional 4 percent provided directly by Medicare and Medicaid. This funding comprised a number of federal resources, including CDC funding and other federal grants, contracts, and cooperative agreements, such as WIC vouchers and Environmental Protection Agency funding. The remainder of funds consisted of state general funds (23 percent), other state or territorial funds (16 percent), other sources of revenue (5 percent), and fees and fines (7 percent) (ASTHO, 2011).

Figure 4-3 shows that on average in 2010, only 23 percent of local health department revenue was derived from federal funding outside of Medicare and Medicaid funding. This 23 percent includes federal funds granted directly to local health departments (6 percent); federal pass-through funds, which are granted to states for dispersal throughout various state programs (14 percent); and ARRA and Public Health Emergency Preparedness (PHEP) grant funding (1 and 2 percent, respectively). The largest single source of local health department revenues was local funding (26 percent) (NACCHO, 2011).

---

[25]This figure varies widely across the states, from 11.2 percent in Wisconsin to 43.8 percent in Arkansas. Fifteen states and the District of Columbia rely on federal grants for less than 20 percent of their annual budgets, while 13 states and Puerto Rico receive more than a third of their income from federal grants (Kaiser Family Foundation, 2010).

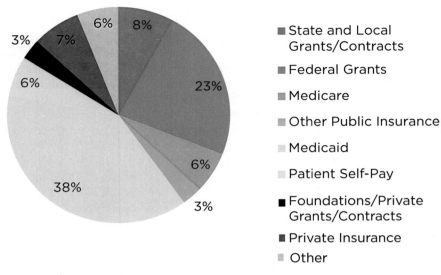

**FIGURE 4-1** Percentage of total annual funding for health centers by revenue source, 2010.
SOURCE: Kaiser Family Foundation, 2010.

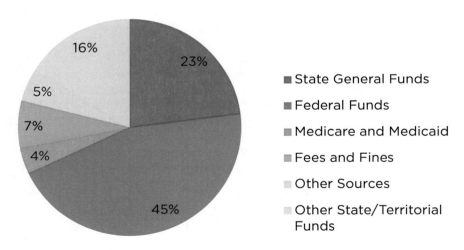

**FIGURE 4-2** Percentage of total annual funding for state health departments by revenue source.
SOURCE: ASTHO, 2011.

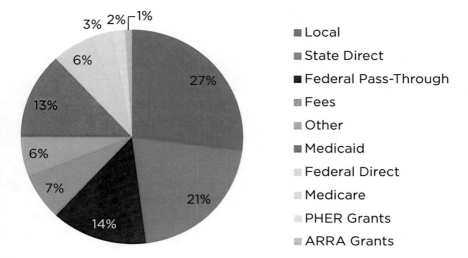

**FIGURE 4-3** Percentage of total annual local health department revenues by revenue source.
NOTE: ARRA = American Recovery and Reinvestment Act; PHER = Public Health and Emergency Response.
SOURCE: NACCHO, 2011.

## Federal Funding Opportunities

Given that HRSA and CDC jointly represent only 1.8 percent of the HHS budget (see Appendix A), it is prudent to look beyond them to other agencies that can assist in funding the integration of primary care and public health. Numerous offices and agencies within HHS have programs designed to promote the health and well-being of individuals, children, families, and communities. Partnering with them could assist HRSA and CDC in fostering integration. For example, the National Institutes of Health (NIH) provides funding for 229 research/disease areas, including cardiovascular disease, colon cancer, stroke, tobacco use, nutrition, and obesity (NIH, 2011). In addition, NIH oversees the Clinical and Translational Science Awards. These awards promote collaboration among diverse sets of stakeholders to identify local health challenges and design practical solutions, and could serve as a mechanism for encouraging integration.

The Social Services Block Grant (SSBG) is one of the most flexible funding sources, providing states with funds for a wide variety of social service and health-related programs. Moreover, up to 10 percent of a state's annual SSBG allotment can be transferred to three health care block grants (the Preventive Health and Health Services Block Grant, the Maternal and

Child Health Services Block Grant, and the Substance Abuse Prevention and Treatment Block Grant) and the Low-Income Home Energy Assistance Program (U.S. House of Representatives Committee on Ways and Means, 2000). Within the Administration for Children and Families is the Community Services Block Grant, which provides services and activities addressing employment, education, housing, nutrition, emergency services, and health (HHS Administration for Children and Families, 2011).

Similarly, CMS oversees programs such as the Children's Health Insurance Program (CHIP), which funds primary care services for children, and the Medicaid program. The Medicaid program pays for health and long-term care services for certain low-income individuals, including children, the elderly, and people with disabilities. States have broad authority to define eligibility, benefits, provider payments, and delivery systems. As a result, Medicaid programs vary widely by state. As mentioned above, CMS also administers the Medicaid Incentives for Prevention of Chronic Disease Program, which provides incentives to Medicaid beneficiaries who participate in prevention programs and demonstrate changes in health risks and outcomes, and the newly created CMMI, which is working on primary care and public health issues.

Finally, the Substance Abuse and Mental Health Services Administration promotes public health for mothers and children through a variety of programs, such as the Substance Abuse Prevention and Treatment Block Grant, the Mental Health Services Block Grant, and the Children's Mental Health Services Program. It also focuses on integrating behavioral health and primary care, as well as reducing the use of tobacco and promoting health and wellness workplace programs.

### Implications of the Current System

In examining the current funding system for primary care and public health, it becomes clear that the system is not well positioned to promote integration. For example, a number of grants from HRSA, CDC, and other agencies are aimed at addressing the same issues, and as a result create overlap on the ground. These competing funding streams have the effect of creating silos at the local level rather than encouraging cooperation across entities. Similarly, as discussed in more detail in Appendix A, funding streams from HRSA and CDC (with the exception of the Preventive Health and Health Services Block Grant) are inflexible. This inflexibility limits what local entities can do with the funds and how they could be used for integration.

Finally, it should be noted that the funds available to HRSA and CDC for supporting and integrating primary care and public health are small compared with what is available to CMS. By joining forces, the three agencies could create much more momentum toward integration.

## REFERENCES

Adashi, E. Y., H. J. Geiger, and M. D. Fine. 2010. Health care reform and primary care—the growing importance of the community health center. *New England Journal of Medicine* 362(22):2047-2050.

AHRQ (Agency for Healthcare Research and Quality). 2010. *Impact infrastructure for maintaining primary care transformation.* http://www.ahrq.gov/research/impactaw.htm (accessed January 31, 2012).

ASTHO (Association of State and Territorial Health Officials). 2011. *ASTHO profile of state public health.* Arlington, VA: ASTHO.

Bell, J., and M. Standish. 2005. Communities and health policy: A pathway for change. *Health Affairs* 24(2):339-342.

Bielaszka-DuVernay, C. 2011. Vermont's blueprint for medical homes, community health teams, and better health at lower cost. *Health Affairs* 30(3):383-386.

Blumenthal, D. 2010. Launching HITECH. *New England Journal of Medicine* 362(5):382-385.

California Department of Public Health. 2010. *Black infant health program.* http://www.cdph.ca.gov/programs/BIH/Pages/default.aspx (accessed February 15, 2012).

Campbell, S., D. Reeves, E. Kontopantelis, E. Middleton, B. Sibbald, and M. Roland. 2007. Quality of primary care in England with the introduction of pay for performance. *New England Journal of Medicine* 357(2):181-190.

Carrier, E., T. Yee, and R. L. Garfield. 2011. *The uninsured and their health care needs: How have they changed since the recession?* The Henry J. Kaiser Family Foundation: Kaiser Commission on Medicaid and the Uninsured.

CBO (Congressional Budget Office). 2006. *Nonprofit hospitals and the provision of community benefits.* Washington, DC: U.S. Congress Congressional Budget Office.

CBO. 2011. *CBO's analysis of the major health care legislation enacted in March 2010: Before the Subcommittee on Health Committee on Energy and Commerce.* Washington, DC: U.S. Congress Congressional Budget Office.

CDC (Centers for Disease Control and Prevention). 2011. *Community transformation grants.* http://www.cdc.gov/communitytransformation/index.htm (accessed November 21, 2011).

CDC. 2012. *Epidemic Intelligence Service (EIS).* http://www.cdc.gov/EIS/index.html (accessed February 10, 2012).

Center for Medicare and Medicaid Innovation. 2011. *Health care innovation challenge.* http://innovations.cms.gov/About/index.html (accessed December 15, 2011).

CMS (Centers for Medicaid & Medicare Services). 2011. *Regulations, guidance & standards.* https://www.cms.gov/home/regsguidance.asp (accessed December 15, 2011).

Dannenberg, A. L., R. Bhatia, B. L. Cole, S. K. Heaton, J. D. Feldman, and C. D. Rutt. 2008. Use of health impact assessment in the U.S. 27 case studies, 1999–2007. *American Journal of Preventive Medicine* 34(3):241-256.

European Centre for Health Policy. 1999. *Health impact assessment: Main concepts and suggested approach.* Brussels: WHO.

Geiger, H. J. 2002. Community-oriented primary care: A path to community development. *American Journal of Public Health* 92(11):1713-1716.

Geiger, H. J. 2005. The first community health centers: A model of enduring value. *Journal of Ambulatory Care Management Community Health Centers' 40th Anniversary Issue* October/December 28(4):313-320.

Grumbach, K., and J. W. Mold. 2009. A health care cooperative extension service. *Journal of the American Medical Association* 301(24):2589-2591.

Gulliford, M. C., M. Ashworth, D. Robotham, and A. Mohiddin. 2007. Achievement of metabolic targets for diabetes by English primary care practices under a new system of incentives. *Diabetic Medicine* 24(5):505-511.

The Henry J. Kaiser Family Foundation. 2011. *Focus on health reform: Summary of new health reform law.* Menlo Park, CA: The Henry J. Kasier Foundation.

HHS (Department of Health and Human Services). 2010. News release: "HHS awards $320 million to expand primary care workforce." http://www.hhs.gov/news/press/2010pres/09/20100927e.html (accessed December 15, 2011).

HHS. 2011. *Prevention and public health fund: Community transformation grants to reduce chronic disease.* http://www.healthcare.gov/news/factsheets/2011/05/grants05132011a.html (accessed February 10, 2012).

HHS Administration for Children and Families. 2011. *Fact sheet.* http://www.acf.hhs.gov/programs/ocs/csbg/aboutus/factsheets.htm (accessed January 16, 2012).

HRSA (Health Resources and Services Administration). 2009. *Accreditation initiative update: Program assistance letter 2009-12.* http://bphc.hrsa.gov/policiesregulations/policies/pal200912.html (accessed December 21, 2011).

HRSA. 2011. *HHS announces new teaching health centers graduate medical education program.* http://www.hrsa.gov/about/news/pressreleases/110125teachinghealthcenters.html (accessed December 15, 2011).

IOM (Institute of Medicine). 2010. *The healthcare imperative: Lowering costs and improving outcomes: Workshop series summary.* Washington, DC: The National Academies Press.

IOM. 2011a. *For the public's health: The role of measurement in action and accountability.* Washington, DC: The National Academies Press.

IOM. 2011b. *For the public's health: Revitalizing law and policy to meet new challenges.* Wahington, DC: The National Academies Press.

IRS (Internal Revenue Service). 2011. Notice 2011-52, notice and request for comments regarding the community health needs assessment requirements for tax-exempt hospitals, edited by IRS. http://www.irs.gov/pub/irs-drop/n-11-52.pdf (accessed November 17, 2011).

Jordan, J., J. Wright, J. Wilkinson, and R. Williams. 1998. Assessing local health needs in primary care: Understanding and experience in three English districts. *Quality Health Care* 7(10180795):83-89.

Kaiser Family Foundation. 2010. *Distribution of revenue by source for federally-funded federally qualified health centers, 2009.* http://www.statehealthfacts.org/comparemaptable.jsp?ind=428&cat=8 (accessed October 24, 2011).

Ku, L., E. Jones, P. Shin, F. R. Byrne, and S. K. Long. 2011. Safety-net providers after health care reform: Lessons from Massachusetts. *Archives of Internal Medicine* 171(15):1379-1384.

MedPAC (Medicare Payment Advisory Commission). 2009. *Accountable care organizations.* Washington, DC: MedPAC.

NACCHO (National Association of County and City Health Officials). 2011. *2010 national profile of local health departments.* Washington, DC: NACCHO.

National Prevention, Health Promotion and Public Health Council. 2011. *National prevention strategy: America's plan for better health and wellness.* Rockville, MD: National Prevention, Health Promotion and Public Health Council.

NIH (National Institutes of Health). 2011. *Estimates of funding for various research, condition, and disease categories (RCDC).* http://report.nih.gov/rcdc/categories/ (accessed November 11, 2011).

NRC (National Research Council). 2011. *Improving health in the United States: The role of health impact assessment.* Washington, DC: The National Academies Press.

Phillips, R. L., S. Bronnikov, S. Petterson, M. Cifuentes, B. Teevan, M. Dodoo, W. D. Pace, and D. R. West. 2011. Case study of a primary care-based accountable care system approach to medical home transformation. *The Journal of Ambulatory Care Management* 34(1):67-77.

Poundstone, K. E., S. A. Strathdee, and D. D. Celentano. 2004. The social epidemiology of human immunodeficiency virus/acquired immunodeficiency syndrome. *Epidemiologic Reviews* 26(1):22-35.

Reynolds, P. P. 2008. A legislative history of federal assistance for health professions training in primary care medicine and dentistry in the United States, 1963-2008. *Academic Medicine* 83(11):1004-1014.

Robert Wood Johnson Foundation, Network for Regional Health Care Improvement, and Pittsburgh Regional Health Initiative. 2009. *From volume to value: Recommendations of the 2008 NRHI healthcare payment reform summit.* Pittsburgh, PA: Network for Regional Healthcare Improvement.

Robinson, J., and R. Elkan. 1996. *Health needs assessment: Theory and practice.* London: Churchill Livingstone.

Roland, M. 2004. Linking physicians' pay to the quality of care—A major experiment in the United Kingdom. *New England Journal of Medicine* 351(14):1448-1454.

Rosenbaum, S., and R. Margulies. 2010. New requirements for tax-exempt charitable hospitals. *Health Reform GPS*, http://www.healthreformgps.org/resources/new-requirements-for-tax-exempt-charitable-hospitals/ (accessed November 16, 2011).

Steele, G. D., J. A. Haynes, D. E. Davis, J. Tomcavage, W. F. Stewart, T. R. Graf, R. A. Paulus, K. Weikel, and J. Shikles. 2010. How Geisinger's advanced medical home model argues the case for rapid-cycle innovation. *Health Affairs* 29(11):2047-2053.

Steinbrook, R. 2009. Health care and the American Recovery and Reinvestment Act. *New England Journal of Medicine* 360(11):1057-1060.

Trust for America's Health. 2011. *Investing in America's health: A state-by-state look at public health funding and key health facts.* Washington, DC: Trust for America's Health.

U.S. House of Representatives Committee on Ways and Means. 2000. Section 10. Title XX Social Services Block Grant program. In *2000 green book background material and data on programs within the jurisdiction of the Committee on Ways and Means.* Washington, DC: U.S. Congress.

U.S. National Archives and Records Administration. 2011. Medicare program; Medicare shared savings program: Accountable care organizations. *Federal Register* 76(212):67802.

Vastag, B. 2004. Donald M. Berwick, MD, MPP advocate for evidence-based health system reform. *Journal of the American Medical Association* 291(16):1945-1947.

Wagner, E. H. 2000. The role of patient care teams in chronic disease management. *British Medical Journal* 320(7234):569-572.

The White House. 2009. *Memorandum for the heads of executive departments and agencies.* http://www.whitehouse.gov/the_press_office/Memorandum-for-the-Heads-of-Executive-Departments-and-Agencies-Subject-Government (accessed November 11, 2011).

WHO (World Health Organization). 2010. *Adelaide statement on Health in All Policies: Moving towards a shared governance for health and well-being.* Geneva, Switzerland: WHO.

# 5

# Conclusions and Recommendations

In approaching its statement of task, the committee reviewed the relevant literature; assessed the current policy context; listened to testimony; engaged in multiple discussions with CDC, HRSA, and other stakeholders; and drew on its members' own experiences. Through this process, the committee reached a number of conclusions about the integration of primary care and public health and formulated five recommendations whose implementation could advance integration to improve population health.

## CONCLUSIONS

The committee developed the following overarching conclusions:

- *The principles identified by the committee in Chapter 2 represent an aspirational yet actionable framework for accelerating progress toward achieving the nation's population health objectives through increased integration of primary care and public health services.*
- *The committee finds that in its current state, the infrastructure for both primary care and public health is inadequate to achieve the nation's population health objectives.*
- *Current patterns of health policy focus and investment lack the alignment necessary to develop an integrated and enduring national infrastructure that can broadly leverage the assets and potential of primary care and public health.*
- *To address this need adequately, agencies both within and outside of the Department of Health and Human Services (HHS) will have*

to *be engaged. The committee notes that there are precedents for this kind of systematic strategy development and investment in national programs, such as the Hill-Burton program to build the nation's hospital infrastructure, investment in the National Institutes of Health and its extramural programs to build the nation's biomedical research infrastructure, and preferential funding for specialty medicine to build high-tech clinical capacity. There has never been an analogous comprehensive and sustained investment in the nation's primary care and public health infrastructure.*

- *While national leadership and prioritization will be needed if the necessary infrastructure is to be built, the committee believes that emerging organizational and funding models for the personal health care delivery system and unprecedented investment in public health and community-based prevention can be leveraged to promote the necessary alignment. However, no single best solution for achieving integration can be prescribed. Community-level application of the framework represented by the principles for integration identified by the committee will require substantial local adaptation and the development of specific structures, relationships, and processes.*

- *Academic health centers often are well positioned to facilitate the integration of primary care and public health and the development of improved means of engagement and integration, as they are often located in communities of need and draw both their patients and their employees from these communities. As illustrated by several of the examples highlighted in Chapter 2, academic health centers can serve as effective partners with both health centers and local health departments in sharing data; aligning clinical, research, and educational programs; and sustaining integrated operations aimed at improving the health of the entire community. Some academic health centers appear to be actively engaged in this role; however, many are not. The evidence in this area is sparse, but the committee believes that creating an interface for the Health Resources and Services Administration (HRSA) and the Centers for Disease Control and Prevention (CDC) to work with academic health centers, their primary care programs, and their local health departments to promote the integration of primary care and public health is an opportunity that should be explored.*

- *The committee believes that a starting point for catalyzing and promoting greater integration of primary care and public health is leveraging existing funds and policy initiatives. Table 4-1 in Chapter 4 highlights opportunities in the Patient Protection and Affordable Care Act (ACA) that HRSA and CDC can exploit for greater integration. Of particular note is the amendment to the Internal*

*Revenue Code that requires local hospitals seeking tax exempt status to conduct community benefit assessments. This effort could be linked with primary care providers and local health departments to build on local expertise and other assessments already under way, forging stronger relationships and encouraging stakeholders to work toward the common goal of improving the community's health.*

## RECOMMENDATIONS

As stated above, the committee regards the principles for integration outlined in Chapter 2 as a framework for action. Implementation of the following recommendations—aimed at the agency and department levels—would assist the leadership of HRSA, CDC, and HHS in creating an environment that would support broader application of these principles.

### Agency Level

**Recommendation 1. To link staff, funds, and data at the regional, state, and local levels, HRSA and CDC should:**

- identify opportunities to coordinate funding streams in selected programs and convene joint staff groups to develop grants, requests for proposals, and metrics for evaluation;
- create an environment in which staff build relationships with each other and local stakeholders by taking full advantage of opportunities to work through the 10 regional HHS offices, state primary care offices and association organizations, state and local health departments, and other mechanisms;
- join efforts to undertake an inventory of existing health and health care databases and identify new data sets, creating from these a consolidated platform for sharing and displaying local population health data that could be used by communities; and
- recognize the need for and commit to developing a trained workforce that can create information systems and make them efficient for the end user.

HRSA and CDC should take a number of leadership actions to encourage local integration efforts. For example, involving representatives from each agency in the development of grants and other funding mechanisms would assist in aligning funds for a common purpose. Likewise, HRSA and CDC should leverage staff at the state, regional, and local levels to promote integration efforts. Either working through health.data.gov, an effort to compile various health data sets, or directly (U.S. Government, 2012), the agencies should commit to convening data experts to undertake a thorough inventory of their databases, identify new data sets, compare the findings, and seek opportunities to consolidate these assets. These efforts should lead to the creation of a consolidated platform for sharing health care and population health data. This platform could ensure that communities can use these data in assessments, intervention planning, and evaluation. The platform would not be "owned" by primary care or public health, but would constitute local neutral space where both sectors could come together to use data that would support the achievement of better health outcomes. The 2011 Institute of Medicine (IOM) report *For the Public's Health: The Role of Measurement in Action and Accountability* provides recommendations that would be relevant to this endeavor. Also needed is a workforce that is trained in developing information systems and making them work for the end user. HRSA and CDC both have a role in the creation of this workforce.

The committee recommends that appropriate incentives to encourage integration be developed at the national level (see Recommendation 5). In some cases, however, such incentives will be developed locally. HRSA and CDC should work with local partners to recognize and learn from these cases.

> **Recommendation 2. To create common research and learning networks to foster and support the integration of primary care and public health to improve population health, HRSA and CDC should:**
>
> - **support the evaluation of existing and the development of new local and regional models of primary care and public health integration, including by working with the Centers for Medicare & Medicaid Services (CMS) Innovation Center (CMMI) on joint evaluations of integration involving Medicare and Medicaid beneficiaries;**
> - **work with the Agency for Healthcare and Research Quality's (AHRQ's) Action Networks on the diffusion of best practices related to the integration of primary care and public health; and**
> - **convene stakeholders at the national and regional levels to share best practices in the integration of primary care and public health.**

Substantial opportunities exist to understand models of successful and sustainable integration taking place in local communities and diffuse that knowledge. Through their role as conveners, HRSA and CDC should take the lead in facilitating a better understanding of the lessons of successful integration from the field. The agencies might consider holding an annual summit; creating a learning collaborative; publishing key findings in various venues, including peer-reviewed journals; and using other mechanisms for sharing findings with stakeholders to foster greater understanding of integration and encourage it at the local, state, and national levels. In addition, the two agencies should work with other agencies, such as the Centers for Medicare & Medicaid Services (CMS) and the Agency for Healthcare Research and Quality (AHRQ), to encourage ongoing evaluation of integration efforts and the diffusion of best practices.

**Recommendation 3. To develop the workforce needed to support the integration of primary care and public health:**

- HRSA and CDC should work with CMS to identify regulatory options for graduate medical education funding that give priority to provider training in primary care and public health settings and specifically support programs that integrate primary care practice with public health.
- HRSA and CDC should explore whether the training component of the Epidemic Intelligence Service (EIS) and the strategic placement of assignees in state and local health departments offer additional opportunities to contribute to the integration of primary care and public health by assisting community health programs supported by HRSA in the use of data for improving community health. Any opportunities identified should be utilized.
- HRSA should create specific Title VII and VIII criteria or preferences related to curriculum development and clinical experiences that favor the integration of primary care and public health.
- HRSA and CDC should create all possible linkages among HRSA's primary care training programs (Title VII and VIII), its public health and preventive medicine training programs, and CDC's public health workforce programs (EIS).
- HRSA and CDC should work together to develop training grants and teaching tools that can prepare the next generation of health professionals for more integrated clinical and public health functions in practice. These tools, which should include a focus on cultural outreach, health education, and nutrition, can be used in the training programs supported by HRSA and CDC, as well as distributed more broadly.

A retooled workforce is one of the most promising ways to model and encourage more complete integration. This retooling will require that primary care providers be educated about public health; that public health workers be educated about primary care; and, most important, that a new cadre of workers who can bridge both sectors in pursuit of improved population health be developed. To achieve significant advances in population health, these efforts must span the life course from preconception through conception, birth, childhood, adolescence, young adulthood, and adulthood and into later life. To this end, joint Title VII/VIII applications could be used to create medicine/nursing workforce training opportunities with the ultimate goal of preparing an integrated workforce capable of working across primary care and public health. In a similar vein, Epidemic Intelligence Service officers could act as a bridge between primary care and public health by helping to transform public health data into information that primary care providers could use at the local level.

### Department Level

Recommendation 4. To improve the integration of primary care and public health through existing HHS programs, as well as newly legislated initiatives, the secretary of HHS should direct:

- CMMI to use its focus on improving community health to support pilots that better integrate primary care and public health and programs in other sectors affecting the broader determinants of health;
- the National Institutes of Health to use the Clinical and Translational Science Awards to encourage the development and diffusion of research advances to applications in the community through primary care and public health;
- the National Committee on Vital and Health Statistics to advise the secretary on integrating policy and incentives for the capture of data that would promote the integration of clinical and public health information;
- the Office of the National Coordinator to consider the development of population measures that would support the integration of community-level clinical and public health data; and
- AHRQ to encourage its Primary Care Extension Program to create linkages between primary care providers and their local health departments.

As stated earlier, the committee believes that current opportunities in the health system could be leveraged to create greater integration of primary care and public health. A number of existing and newly created programs could be used as a starting point for strengthening integration, and the committee encourages the secretary of HHS to take full advantage of these opportunities. While the above list is not complete, the committee believes it could be used to begin the effort, but also urges the secretary to look for other opportunities.

> **Recommendation 5. The secretary of HHS should work with all agencies within the department as a first step in the development of a national strategy and investment plan for the creation of a primary care and public health infrastructure strong enough and appropriately integrated to enable the agencies to play their appropriate roles in furthering the nation's population health goals.**

By engaging HHS agencies to work together in creating an infrastructure to facilitate the integration of primary care and public health, the secretary could create momentum around this topic. To achieve a truly national strategy and infrastructure, however, agencies beyond HHS should be involved. The National Prevention, Health Promotion and Public Health Council, chaired by the Surgeon General, could undertake this task. Alternatively, the Domestic Policy Council, which is currently leading the Obama administration's policy on place-based initiatives, could be engaged on this topic.

To improve the population's health and meet national health goals, such as those of Healthy People 2020, the committee encourages the secretary to explore ways of leveraging funding through existing programs, pool existing resources, and create incentives that will encourage a willingness to integrate among local stakeholders.

## BROADER OPPORTUNITIES FOR INTEGRATION

While its task was to assist HRSA and CDC in identifying opportunities to integrate primary care and public health, the committee believes it would be remiss if it failed to note some broader opportunities for integration. Although the opportunities touched on below are not the focus of this report, the committee encourages those working in primary care and public health to explore them.

The patient-centered medical home, discussed in Chapter 4, has been endorsed by primary care providers and others (American Academy of Family Physicians et al., 2007; IOM, 2010; National Partnership for Women & Families, 2012). As a model that emphasizes care coordination facilitated by increased data sharing, as well as the role of the patient's family and community, it provides a clear-cut opportunity for integrating primary care and public health. Given the provisions in the ACA that promote the expansion of the patient-centered medical home concept for Medicaid patients, more primary care practices are expected to move toward this model. As they do so, health departments could be poised to work with them, diffusing the benefits of care coordination into the community.

Another opportunity created in the ACA, and discussed in Chapter 4, is accountable care organizations (ACOs), groups of hospitals and clinicians that work together to provide care for a panel of Medicare beneficiaries (at least 5,000). While the role of ACOs is to provide primary care and other health care services, partnering with health departments would broaden the range of services available to the patient panel. As the first ACOs begin operating in 2012, they should reach out to health departments to forge links to community programs and public health services.

Employer groups provide another opportunity for integration. Businesses are increasingly concerned about the health of their own workers and their social responsibility in the communities in which they are located and in which their markets exist. The National Business Group on Health and regional groups such as the Pacific Business Group on Health and the Midwest Business Group on Health are active in developing initiatives in which businesses can contribute to local community health. Primary care providers could have a role in working with these groups.

While health departments have responsibility for providing public health services in most places in the United States, they do not exist in some places. In those cases, public health services are provided by other entities, such as community organizations or academic health centers. Primary care groups should consider partnering with these entities in places that lack formal health departments.

Finally, two large-scale policy initiatives could support integration: the place-based initiatives supported by the White House and the National Prevention Strategy issued by the National Prevention, Health Promotion and Public Health Council. As discussed in Chapter 4, place-based initiatives focus resources in areas such as economic development, transportation, education, or health promotion to create coordinated action. Coordination of the delivery of these resources creates alignment that impacts the community as a whole. The emphasis of these initiatives on local communities echoes the principles necessary for integration. Through its implementation, this policy could encourage primary care and public health to work together to improve population health. The National Prevention Strategy is an integrated national strategy designed to improve the health of the nation by encouraging partnerships among government entities, businesses, community-based organizations, individuals, and others. With its focus in four areas—healthy communities, clinical and community preventive services, empowered people, and the elimination of health disparities—the strategy aligns closely with the principles for integration. This strategy also could serve as a catalyst for promoting the integration of primary care and public health.

These final two policy examples represent the type of broad, intersectoral collaboration that is necessary to realize significant, sustained improvements in population health. Through an improved understanding of the broad determinants of health, it has become abundantly clear that a wide array of public and private actors contribute directly or indirectly to the health outcomes of the nation's population. By establishing a unified focus on health, these actors can work with one another to produce a greater impact than any could achieve on its own. With explicit missions to foster healthy populations, primary care and public health have critical roles in population health. Through integration, both sectors can increase their capacity to directly improve the health and health care of people in communities nationwide. And by linking with other organizations, institutions, and community resources, the leadership of primary care and public health can set the pace for interdisciplinary, intersectoral cooperation and help establish a national focus on the health of communities.

## REFERENCES

American Academy of Family Physicians, American Academy of Pediatrics, American College of Physicians, and American Osteopathic Association. 2007. *Joint principles of the patient-centered medical home*. http://www.pcpcc.net/content/joint-principles-patient-centered-medical-home (accessed December 15, 2011).

IOM (Institute of Medicine). 2010. *The future of nursing: Leading change, advancing health*. Washington, DC: The National Academies Press.

IOM. 2011. *For the public's health: The role of measurement in action and accountability*. Washington, DC: The National Academies Press.

National Partnership for Women & Families. 2012. *National Partnership for Women & Families*. 2012. http://www.nationalpartnership.org/site/PageServer (accessed February 14, 2012).

U.S. Government. 2012. *Health data community*. http://www.data.gov/health (accessed February 14, 2012).

# Appendix A

# Health Resources and Services Administration (HRSA) and Centers for Disease Control and Prevention (CDC)

In recent years, the Health Resources and Services Administration (HRSA) and the Centers for Disease Control and Prevention (CDC) have articulated a vision of how their work can impact the broader determinants of health (Frieden, 2010; HRSA, 2010). To understand how this work can be accomplished within and between the agencies, it is important to understand the current organization of each agency and how funding flows into and through their networks. This appendix provides a brief overview of each agency and reviews their macro-level funding streams as they relate to primary care and public health opportunities.

## WITHIN THE CONTEXT OF THE DEPARTMENT OF HEALTH AND HUMAN SERVICES

The Department of Health and Human Services (HHS) is the principal agency charged with protecting the health of all Americans, and in fiscal year 2010, it spent $854 billion in pursuit of that goal (see Table A-1 for details). It is notable that together, HRSA and CDC account for less than 2 percent of the department's budget. In contrast, the National Institutes of Health accounts for 3.65 percent of the HHS budget, the Administration for Children and Families for 6.1 percent, and the Centers for Medicare & Medicaid Services (CMS) for fully 86.5 percent (HHS, 2011).

While HRSA and CDC operate on less than 0.5 percent of total federal outlays , they are responsible for the provision of primary care for tens of millions of vulnerable individuals and for oversight of the public health of the nation, respectively, and thus are positioned to facilitate the integration

**TABLE A-1** HHS Outlays by Operating Division (Fiscal Year 2010)

| Operating Division | Outlays (in millions of $) | Percentage of Total Outlays |
|---|---|---|
| Centers for Medicare & Medicaid Services | 732,896 | 85.80 |
| Administration for Children and Families | 56,370 | 6.60 |
| National Institutes of Health | 33,052 | 3.87 |
| Health Resources and Services Administration | 8,569 | 1.00 |
| Centers for Disease Control and Prevention | 6,957 | 0.81 |
| Public Health and Social Services Emergency Fund | 4,890 | 0.57 |
| Indian Health Service | 4,350 | 0.51 |
| Substance Abuse and Mental Health Services | 3,325 | 0.39 |
| Food and Drug Administration | 2,117 | 0.25 |
| Administration on Aging | 1,512 | 0.18 |
| Program Support Center | 575 | 0.07 |
| Departmental Management | 497 | 0.06 |
| Agency for Healthcare Research and Quality | 80 | 0.01 |
| Office of the National Coordinator | 115 | 0.01 |
| Medicare Hearings and Appeals | 64 | 0.01 |
| Office of Inspector General | 91 | 0.01 |
| Office for Civil Rights | 34 | 0.00 |
| Prevention and Wellness | 10 | 0.00 |
| Health Insurance Reform Implementation Fund | 21 | 0.00 |
| World Trade Center Health Program Fund | 0 | 0.00 |
| Offsetting Collections | −1,351 | −0.16 |
| Total Health and Human Services | 854,174 | 100.00 |

SOURCE: HHS, 2011.

of primary care and public health. Yet, while they share certain objectives, HRSA and CDC are two very different agencies, and located more than 600 miles apart; they have very different responsibilities for fostering the health of the U.S. population.

Among HHS agencies, HRSA and CDC have especially important roles to play in improving population health. HRSA plays a strategic role in helping to ensure access to health services for uninsured and vulnerable populations. Among its other activities, it provides funding to support the provision of primary care services at community health centers, Ryan White clinics, and rural health clinics, as well as training programs for the primary care workforce and maternal and child health care programs. And with its focus on health promotion, prevention, and preparedness, CDC is recognized as a global leader in public health. The agency works with local and state health departments on a number of efforts, including implementing disease surveillance systems, preventing and controlling infectious and chronic diseases, reducing injuries, eliminating workplace hazards, and addressing environmental health threats. This appendix examines HRSA and CDC in greater detail.

## HEALTH RESOURCES AND SERVICES ADMINISTRATION

Established in 1980, HRSA is the primary federal agency responsible for ensuring access to health care services for people who are uninsured, isolated, or medically vulnerable, including those living with HIV/AIDS, mothers and children, and those living in rural areas. HRSA's vision is "Healthy Communities, Healthy People," and its mission is "to improve health and achieve health equity through access to quality services, a skilled health workforce and innovative programs" (HRSA, 2011a). HRSA has established four goals to help achieve its vision and mission: to improve (1) access to quality care and services, (2) the health workforce, (3) healthy communities, and (4) health equity (HRSA, 2011a).

At its highest level, HRSA is organized into 6 bureaus and 10 offices (Figure A-1) (HRSA, 2011c). Each bureau provides clinical and preventive services to vulnerable populations. For instance, the Bureau of Primary Health Care funds health centers in underserved communities that provide comprehensive primary and preventive health care for medically under-served populations regardless of their ability to pay (HRSA, 2011b), while the Maternal and Child Health Bureau functions to improve the health of mothers, infants, and children and aims to reduce health disparities relat-ing to such issues as infant mortality, access to pre- and postnatal care, and health care for children with special health care needs (HRSA, 2011d).

Among other efforts, HRSA functions to improve health by funding health care initiatives and systems such as health clinics, maternal and child health initiatives, and workforce programs including training and loan reimbursement programs. HRSA supports 70 programs that provide funding to such entities as academic institutions, community health centers, public health departments, and local communities. HRSA programs and their funding share some key features. HRSA programs include few flex-ible funding sources and include only one block grant—the Maternal and Child Health Block Grant. In contrast with the CDC programs discussed below, 10 of the HRSA programs allocate funds based on a formula, and 12 of the HRSA project grants are funded through cooperative agreements which allows HRSA to be substantially involved in local activities. Despite this variability, the majority of HRSA awards are project grants designated for a specified use or project (Federal Funds Information for States, 2011).

Additionally, HRSA programs have some specific funding restrictions. Fifteen of the programs impose some type of matching requirement, and 22 have a maintenance-of-effort provision. These may require that additional

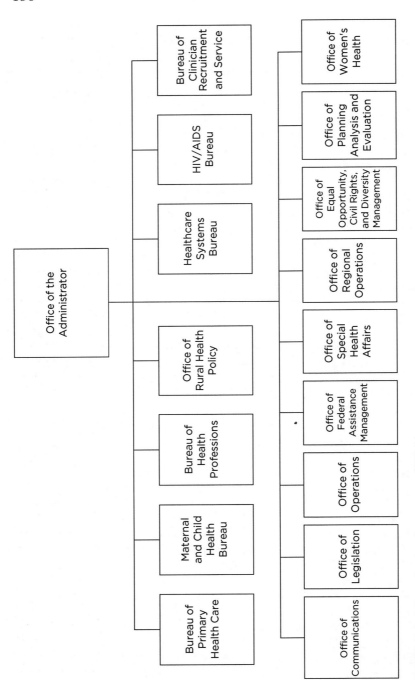

**FIGURE A-1** Organizational structure of HRSA.
SOURCE: HRSA, 2011c.

**TABLE A-2** HRSA Fiscal Year 2010 Budget Authority

| Activity | Funding Level (in millions of $) | Percent of Total |
|---|---|---|
| HIV/AIDS | 2,315 | 30.90 |
| Primary Care | 2,253 | 30.07 |
| Health Workforce | 1,230 | 16.42 |
| Maternal and Child Health | 984 | 13.13 |
| Other Activities | 837 | 11.17 |
| Health Care Systems | 267 | 3.56 |
| Rural Health | 185 | 2.47 |
| Less Funds from Other Sources | –579 | –7.73 |
| TOTAL | 7,492 | 100.00 |

SOURCE: HHS, 2011.

funds be generated by the program or through other grants. Many of these programs have a supplantation provision requiring that the grantee use the funds to supplement, not supplant, existing funding for specified grant activities. These provisions are in addition to funding restrictions, such as on the use of funds for the delivery of health care services, indirect costs, and facility construction (Federal Funds Information for States, 2011).

In fiscal year 2010, HRSA was appropriated $7.5 billion (Table A-2). It received nearly equal funding for its HIV/AIDS and primary care initiatives (30.9 and 30.1 percent, respectively), while 16 percent of its funding was dedicated to health workforce development and maintenance (HHS, 2011).

## CENTERS FOR DISEASE CONTROL AND PREVENTION

Established in 1942, CDC is perhaps the most well known of Department of Health and Human Services (HHS) agencies. The agency pursues its mission of "Health Protection ... Health Equity" through collaboration with nationwide and global partners to "monitor health, detect and investigate health problems, conduct research to enhance prevention, develop and advocate sound public health policies, implement prevention strategies, promote healthy behaviors, foster safe and healthful environments, and provide leadership and training" (CDC, 2010).

At its highest level, CDC is organized into five offices, the Center for Global Health, and the National Institute for Occupational Safety and Health (Figure A-2). Three of these offices—the Office of Infectious Diseases; the Office of Noncommunicable Disease, Injury, and Environmental Health; and the Office of Surveillance, Epidemiology and Laboratory Services—are further divided into national centers and program offices (CDC, 2011b). These centers and offices are further partitioned into divisions

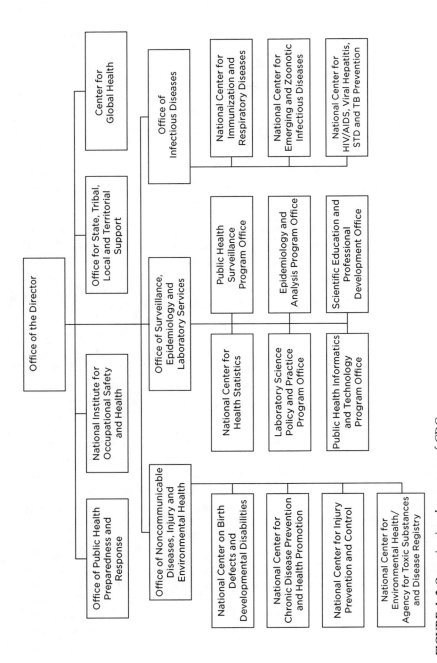

**FIGURE A-2** Organizational structure of CDC.
SOURCE: CDC, 2011b.

and then branches, which are narrowly focused on health topic areas. For instance, the National Center for Chronic Disease Prevention and Health Promotion comprises nine divisions: the Division of Adolescent and School Health; the Division of Cancer Prevention and Control; the Division of Adult and Community Health; the Division of Diabetes Translation; the Division of Nutrition, Physical Activity and Obesity; the Division of Reproductive Health; the Office of Smoking and Health; the Division for Heart Disease and Stroke Prevention; and the Division of Oral Health (CDC, 2011a). Each division, center, and office is headed by a director who ultimately reports to the director of CDC and the secretary of HHS.

CDC functions to improve the health of all Americans through various public health initiatives, such as vaccine promotion, infectious disease prevention, and management of chronic disease. While organizing many of its own campaigns, CDC functions largely through its grant-making programs. These programs cover a broad spectrum and share several features. Only one program—the Preventive Health and Health Services Block Grant—provides flexible funding to states that can be used for a variety of activities, from clinical services to data surveillance. The remaining CDC programs provide funding through project grants, whereby the funding is competitive and restricted to a specified use or project. Twenty-nine of these project grants operate as cooperative agreements between the federal government and recipient(s) (Federal Funds Information for States, 2011).

Programs in the CDC inventory also are similar in their funding restrictions. Most have general restrictions that apply to all CDC grants. These restrictions generally entail use limitations, which allow funding only for reasonable program costs and exclude the use of funds for the purchase of equipment and construction and for rehabilitative services or clinical care. These restrictions also require the recipient to play a substantial role in carrying out the project objectives and do not allow for the reimbursement of pre-award costs. In addition to these general restrictions, some programs impose matching or maintenance-of-effort requirements. For example, state health departments must match $1 for every $4 they receive under cooperative agreements for state-based diabetes control programs and evaluation of surveillance systems. Additionally, while some programs have specific maintenance-of-effort requirements, others have supplantation provisions (Federal Funds Information for States, 2011).

In fiscal year 2010, CDC was appropriated nearly $6.5 billion in discretionary funds (Table A-3). At 23.5 percent, the largest portion of this funding was dedicated to public health preparedness and response. This was followed by funding for prevention of HIV/AIDS, viral hepatitis, sexually transmitted diseases (STDs), and tuberculosis (17.3 percent) and $949 million for chronic disease prevention and health promotion (HHS, 2011). The primary uses of these funds are to support public health through state

**TABLE A-3** CDC Fiscal Year 2010 Budget Authority

| Activity | Funding Level (in millions of $) | Percent of Total |
|---|---|---|
| Public Health Preparedness and Response | 1,522 | 23.51 |
| HIV/AIDS, Viral Hepatitis, STD, and TB Prevention | 1,119 | 17.28 |
| Chronic Disease Prevention and Health Promotion | 949 | 14.66 |
| Immunization and Respiratory Diseases | 721 | 11.14 |
| Public Health Scientific Services | 441 | 6.81 |
| Occupational Safety and Health | 430 | 6.64 |
| Business Support Services | 367 | 5.67 |
| Global Health | 354 | 5.47 |
| Emerging and Zoonotic Infectious Diseases | 281 | 4.34 |
| Public Health Leadership and Support | 194 | 3.00 |
| Environmental Health | 181 | 2.80 |
| Injury Prevention and Control | 149 | 2.30 |
| Child Health, Disabilities, and Blood Disorders | 144 | 2.22 |
| Preventive Health and Health Services Block Grant | 100 | 1.54 |
| Agency for Toxic Substances and Disease Registry | 100 | 1.54 |
| Buildings and Facilities | 69 | 1.07 |
| User Fees | 2 | 0.03 |
| Less Funds from Other Sources | −649 | −10.02 |
| TOTAL | 6,474 | 100.00 |

NOTE: STD = sexually transmitted disease; TB = tuberculosis.
SOURCE: HHS, 2011.

and local health departments and to sponsor nationwide public health research and programming.

## REFERENCES

CDC (Centers for Disease Control and Prevention). 2010. *About CDC: Vision, mission, core values, and pledge.* http://www.cdc.gov/about/organization/mission.htm (accessed November 1, 2011).

CDC. 2011a. *Chronic disease prevention and health promotion: Organizational chart.* http://www.cdc.gov/chronicdisease/about/org_chart.htm (accessed November 1, 2011).

CDC. 2011b. *Department of Health and Human Services Centers for Disease Control and Prevention (CDC).* http://www.cdc.gov/maso/pdf/CDC_Chart_wNames.pdf (accessed November 1, 2011).

Federal Funds Information for States. 2011 (unpublished). *Inventory of federal funding streams: A detailed review of HRSA and CDC funds.* Washington, DC: Institute of Medicine.

Frieden, T. R. 2010. A framework for public health action: The health impact pyramid. *American Journal of Public Health* 100(4):590-595.

HHS (Department of Health and Human Services). 2011. *Advancing the health, safety, and well-being of our people: FY 2012 president's budget for HHS.* Washington, DC: HHS.

HRSA (Health Resources and Services Administration). 2010. *Public Health Steering Committee recommendations (draft).* Washington, DC: HRSA.

HRSA. 2011a. *About HRSA.* http://www.hrsa.gov/about/index.html (accessed November 1, 2011).

HRSA. 2011b. *Bureau of Primary Health Care.* http://www.hrsa.gov/about/organization/bureaus/bphc/index.html (accessed November 1, 2011).

HRSA. 2011c. *Bureaus and offices.* http://www.hrsa.gov/about/organization/bureaus/index.html (accessed November 1, 2011).

HRSA. 2011d. *Maternal and Child Health Bureau.* http://www.hrsa.gov/about/organization/bureaus/mchb/index.html (accessed November 1, 2011).

# Appendix B

# HRSA-Supported Primary Care Systems and Health Departments

The statement of task directed the committee to explicitly consider HRSA-supported primary care systems and health departments. This appendix provides an overview of these entities.

## HRSA-SUPPORTED PRIMARY CARE SYSTEMS

While most primary care in the United States is delivered outside of HRSA-supported primary care systems, these systems served 19.5 million patients in 2010 (HRSA, 2011j) and play a critical strategic role in addressing health disparities. The most widely recognized of these primary care systems are the health centers funded under the Health Center Program or designated as federally qualified health center (FQHC) look-alikes. These centers are community-based and patient-directed organizations that provide comprehensive primary care and preventive services in medically underserved communities for vulnerable populations with limited access to health care. In addition, HRSA supports other primary care systems as well.

### Health Centers

HRSA supports two classes of health centers (HRSA, 2011k). The first are Health Center Program grantees or federally funded health centers. These are public and private nonprofit health care organizations that meet certain criteria under the Medicare and Medicaid programs (Sections 1861[(aa)][(4)] and 1905[(l)][(2)][(B)], respectively, of the Social Security Act) and receive funds under Section 330 of the Public Health

Service Act. They include community health centers, migrant health centers, Healthcare for the Homeless centers, and Public Housing Primary Care centers. These health centers are required to report administrative, clinical, and other information to the Bureau of Primary Health Care within HRSA.

The second class of health center comprises federally qualified health center (FQHC) look-alikes, health centers that do not receive grant funding under Section 330 but have been identified by HRSA and certified by the Centers for Medicare & Medicaid Services (CMS) as meeting Section 330 requirements. Although FQHC look-alikes do not receive Section 330 funding, they report to the Bureau of Primary Health Care and are eligible for other FQHC[1] benefits through CMS.

As mentioned in Chapter 3, this report uses the term "health center" to refer to Health Center Program grantees and FQHC look-alike organizations. The term does not refer to FQHCs that are sponsored by tribal or urban Indian health organizations, except for those that receive Health Center Program grants.

All HRSA-supported health centers are required to meet certain criteria to maintain their health center designation. Health centers must meet performance and accountability requirements established by HRSA. They must be governed by a community board, at least 51 percent of whose members represent the population served by the center. Additionally, health centers must provide comprehensive primary health care and supportive services and use a sliding-scale system to charge patients without health insurance. These services include well-child care, nutritional assessment and referral services, blood pressure and weight management, clinical breast examination, and prenatal services. Most important, health centers must be located in a medically underserved area or serve a specified medically underserved population (HRSA, 2011b).

Migrant health centers are a strong example of health centers that serve a medically underserved population, focusing on communities of migrant and seasonal farm workers who face unique health care challenges. These challenges may be due to a relatively small number of individuals requiring care over a large geographic area, the transient nature of migrant and seasonal farm work, and/or the inability of existing health centers to handle the cyclical nature of seasonal work and the influx and outflow of patients. Approximately 90 percent of migrant health centers are funded as Health Center Program grantees serving special populations; the remaining 10 per-

---

[1] The term FQHC is a designation determined and used by CMS to indicate that an entity can be reimbursed using specific methodologies statutorily designed for FQHCs. Here the term FQHC is used to indicate these CMS-designated entities, and includes designated Health Center Program grantees, FQHC look-alikes, and outpatient health clinics associated with tribal or urban Indian health organizations that are not administered or overseen by HRSA.

cent operate under migrant health voucher programs in which primary care services for migrant workers are subcontracted to existing local providers (National Center for Farmworker Health, 2011a,b).

FQHCs (and rural health clinics, described next) are reimbursed by Medicare through a Prospective Payment System (PPS). This system establishes a fee to be paid to the provider regardless of the service rendered, and is designed to encourage comprehensive care. There is no limit on the number of visits each patient can make per year. The reimbursement is based on yearly cost reports, which take into account the overall cost of operations relative to clinical production. Medicare and Medicaid PPS rates are set by the respective agencies but are generally similar.

In 2010, 1,124 health centers served more than 19 million patients. Approximately one-third of these patients were individuals aged 18 or younger, 7.3 million were uninsured, and nearly 863,000 were migrant or seasonal farm workers and their families (HRSA, 2011j). Table B-1 presents more detailed information on health centers.

**TABLE B-1** Snapshot of Health Centers

| Characteristic | Number | Percentage |
|---|---|---|
| Total Patients | 19,469,467 | |
| | | |
| Patients by Age | | |
| Children (<18) | 6,251,866 | 32.11 |
| Adults (18-64) | 11,885,206 | 61.05 |
| Geriatric patients (65 and over) | 1,332,395 | 6.84 |
| | | |
| Number of Patients by Insurance Status | | |
| Uninsured | 7,308,655 | 37.54 |
| Uninsured children (0-19) | 1,393,640 | 7.16 |
| Medicaid/CHIP | 7,505,047 | 38.55 |
| Medicare | 1,461,485 | 7.51 |
| Other third party | 2,699,183 | 13.86 |
| | | |
| Patients below the poverty level | 10,726,964 | 55.10 |
| | | |
| Staffing | | |
| Total staff | 131,660.23 | |
| Primary care physicians | 9,592.10 | |
| Nurse practitioners | 3,807.86 | |
| Physician assistants | 2,034.20 | |
| Certified nurse midwives | 520.28 | |
| Dentists | 2,881.89 | |

NOTE: CHIP = Children's Health Insurance Program.
SOURCE: HRSA, 2011j.

## Rural Health Clinics

Another HRSA-supported clinical service is the rural health clinic program, initiated to increase primary care services for Medicaid and Medicare patients in rural communities. As of August 2011, more than 3,800 rural health clinics were in operation across the United States, with 28 states containing more than 50 such centers (CMS Rural Health Center, 2011).

Rural health clinics must meet certain criteria to maintain their rural health clinic designation. They must be located in a nonurbanized medically underserved or health professional shortage area. They must utilize a team of physicians and other practitioners, such as nurse practitioners, physician assistants, and certified nurse midwives, and must be staffed at least 50 percent of the time by nonphysician practitioners. Rural health clinics are not required to provide any preventive health, preventive dental health, or case management services. The scope of their services is limited to emergency care; outpatient primary care; and basic laboratory services such as urine testing by stick or tablet, blood sugar tests, and the collection of cultures for transmittal to a certified laboratory for analysis (HRSA, 2006).

## Disease-Specific Health Centers

HRSA supports a number of disease-specific health centers. These centers focus on serving populations with particular diseases or areas with concentrated rates of a particular disease resulting from geographic proximity to exposures and other factors. The most renowned of these centers are Ryan White clinics, which exist as a part of the Ryan White Program. That program, the largest federal program focused exclusively on HIV/AIDS care, was designed to increase federal funding for centers providing primary care to HIV/AIDS patient (HRSA, 2011a).

The Ryan White Program has six parts. Part A funds are used to provide care for people living with HIV, including outpatient and ambulatory medical care, oral health care, mental health services, substance abuse outpatient care, and assistance with health insurance premiums and cost sharing for low-income individuals (HRSA, 2011e). Part B provides grants to states and U.S. territories to improve the quality, availability, and organization of HIV/AIDS health care and support services (HRSA, 2011f). Part C gives grants directly to service providers to support outpatient HIV early intervention services, and provide primary care and ambulatory care (HRSA, 2011g). Part D focuses on services to families and awards funds to public and private organizations for such activities as community outreach, prevention programs, primary and specialty medical care, and psychosocial services. It also supports efforts to improve access to clinical trials and research for vulnerable populations (HRSA, 2011h). Finally, Part F provides funds for a variety of programs, including the Special Projects of National Significance Program, the AIDS Education and Training Centers Program, dental programs, and the Minority AIDS Initiative (HRSA, 2011i). In 2010, the Ryan White Program was funded at approximately $2.2 billion (HRSA, 2011d).

## Local Variability

Like local health departments (discussed below), HRSA-supported primary care systems vary widely. Health centers and rural health clinics serve a variety of populations and population sizes. Nationally, for example, health centers serve an average of 2,416 patients per center site; however, this number varies from 488 patients per site in Alaska to 3,408 patients per site in Washington state and 5,972 patients per site in the U.S. territory of Puerto Rico (National Association of Community Health Centers, 2011). This variability results from a number of factors, including the size of the overall population and the geographic distribution of both the general and underserved populations, the degree of stability of these populations, the number and location of the centers, and the presence of alternative sources of care in the community.

While health centers may vary from program to program, there is some standardization for entities within each funding program. As noted earlier, for instance, rural health clinics must meet a number of requirements to receive that designation. These requirements not only set minimum service levels, but also include services that these clinics cannot provide using program funds. Additional sources of funding may impose further requirements or allow centers to provide additional services. For example, some centers may be associated with academic institutions and may use the center as a teaching environment for medical interns and residents. These centers may provide expanded services using institutional funding. The presence of auxiliary staff, such as social workers, mental health and substance abuse personnel, and community health workers,[2] varies from center to center as well.

## HEALTH DEPARTMENTS

Health departments have primary responsibility for the provision of essential public health services. The governmental public health system, embodied in health departments, evolved in response to the hunger, malnu-

---

[2]A community health worker is defined as a person who links members of the community to health services. The designation encompasses *promotores de salud* (community health workers in Spanish) and patient navigators (who work with specific patients), as well as other terms.

trition, scurvy, and infectious diseases that were epidemic in the American colonies. Early public health interventions often were based in policy, with colonies enacting laws to regulate waste disposal and the quarantining of ships. Smallpox inoculation was another early demonstration of the effectiveness of public health interventions, dramatically reducing the mortality rate from that disease among the vaccinated (Novick and Mays, 2005).

Since the colonial period, health departments have evolved to meet the public's changing needs and grown in influence. Currently, federal health agencies can set a national health policy agenda and steer the system by allocating resources across the designated priorities. While national agendas are set at the federal level, states play a pivotal role in the system, often acting as intermediaries between the federal government and local municipalities (Novick and Mays, 2005). Local health departments often are the primary entities implementing public health activities in local communities.

## State Health Departments

State health departments provide essential expertise and other support for local public health departments and in 26 states act as the local public health department for some or all of their state's communities. These health departments are responsible for the state's public health—including preventive, protective, and wellness services—and the allocation of public health resources according to local needs.

### Structure and Governance

Some state health departments are independent organizations, while others operate within an umbrella agency that is also responsible for such functions as Medicaid, services for the elderly, and public assistance (ASTHO, 2011a). Public health agencies are more likely to be independent in states with larger populations: this is the case in 71 percent of states with medium-sized populations and 65 percent of those with large populations (ASTHO, 2011a).

Governance relationships between state and local agencies vary, and these variations affect the way public health services are delivered. In 14 states, governance is wholly or largely centralized such that the state government has primary responsibility for leading local agencies, including decision-making authority in most matters related to budget, the issuance of public health orders, and the appointment of local health officials. In five states, a shared governance model is used whereby either local or state governments may lead local agencies, with responsibility for decisions regarding budget, the issuance of public health orders, and the appointment of local health officials (ASTHO, 2011a). Finally, 27 states have a governance structure that is wholly or largely decentralized. Mainly local employees lead the local agencies, and local governments have some decision-making authority.

## Expenditures and Revenues

For fiscal year (FY) 2009, state health department revenues were reported for 48 states; they totaled $31.5 billion. If revenues are estimated for the two remaining states and the District of Columbia, the total is about $34 billion. State health department revenues come from federal sources (45 percent); state general funds (23 percent); other state funds (16 percent); fees and fines (7 percent); Medicare and Medicaid (4 percent); and other sources (5 percent), such as tobacco settlement funds, payment for direct clinical services (other than Medicare and Medicaid), foundations, and other private donations. Average revenue per capita was $126 in FY 2009 (ASTHO, 2011a).

Total state health department expenditures for FY 2009 for the 48 states for which data are available were $22.5 billion. If revenues are estimated for the two states without expenditure data and the District of Columbia, the total is about $25 billion. Almost half of these expenditures were for either the Special Supplemental Nutrition Program for Women, Infants, and Children (WIC) (24 percent of the total) or improving consumer health (also 24 percent), a category that includes access to care programs and direct clinical services, such as tuberculosis treatment, adult day care, early childhood programs, and local health clinics. Thirteen percent of state health department expenditures were for infectious disease programming, while 8 percent was dedicated to chronic disease prevention. Six percent went to improving the quality of health care and 5 percent to each of the following: all-hazards preparedness, environmental protection, administration, and other. A small portion was spent on health laboratories (2 percent), injury prevention (2 percent), health data (1 percent), and vital statistics (1 percent) (ASTHO, 2011a).

## Workforce

In 2010, state (including the District of Columbia) health departments were estimated to have about 107,000 full-time employees. Of these, more than 27,000 were assigned to local health departments and another 17,000 to regional or district offices. The greatest numbers of these employees were administrative and clerical personnel, followed by public health nurses. On average, state health departments had about 288 vacant positions but were recruiting for only about 15 percent of these—likely as a result of hiring freezes in many states (87 percent of states have had such a freeze in effect since 2008).

As one would expect, state health departments serving larger populations employed larger numbers of full-time equivalents. The average number of employees in the state health departments serving the smallest populations was 876, while those serving midsized populations had an average of 2,045 employees and those serving the largest populations an average of 3,537. Considered on a per capita basis, smaller states employed more staff: 82 per 100,000 persons, compared with 47 for midsized states and 27 for large states (ASTHO, 2011b).

### Priorities and Responsibilities

Top priorities cited by state health leaders included improving infrastructure and increasing capacity in terms of technology and workforce capacity (17 percent of states); quality improvement (9 percent); health promotion and prevention (8 percent); obesity, nutrition, and physical activity (6 percent); and emergency preparedness (6 percent). Responsibilities of state health departments included vaccine order management and inventory distribution, behavioral risk factor surveillance, reportable diseases, vital statistics, and testing of likely bioterrorism agents (ASTHO, 2011a).

### Local Health Departments

Local health departments are formed at the discretion of the state or local jurisdiction and often perform a broad range of services depending on the jurisdiction. To address some of this variability, in 2005 the National Association of County and City Health Officials (NACCHO) led the development of the "Operational Definition of a Functional Local Health Department" (NACCHO, 2005). This definition identifies the essential functions a citizen should expect a state, local, tribal, or territorial health department to perform. Furthermore, standards for local public health have been established, and voluntary accreditation for local health departments started in 2011. The Public Health Accreditation Board, a national nonprofit organization, based the public health standards on the 10 essential public health services (see Box 1-2 in Chapter 1) and the NACCHO definition. This accreditation is endorsed by NACCHO and is encouraged as a way of ensuring consistent and quality local public health services for all communities across the United States. Nonetheless, great variability remains among local health departments in terms of population size served, jurisdiction, and governance; expenditures and revenues; workforce; role and scope of services; and information technology.

*Population Size, Jurisdiction, and Governance*

The majority of local health departments serve small populations. Approximately 63 percent serve fewer than 50,000 people, and only 5 percent serve 500,000 or more. The population size served often is governed by the department's geographic jurisdiction. In 2010, 68 percent of health departments served county systems, 21 percent served cities or towns, 8 percent served multiple counties, and 4 percent served multiple cities or a county and a city located outside of the county line (NACCHO, 2011a). Many health departments (75 percent) also are associated with one or more local boards of health, which serve to represent local perspectives and needs, institute public health regulations, set and impose fees, and administer other activities (NACCHO, 2011a).

*Expenditures and Revenues*

Local health departments vary greatly in their expenditures and revenues. According to NACCHO's 2010 National Profile (NACCHO, 2011a), roughly one-third of all local health departments had total expenditures of less than $1 million, another third had expenditures of $1-$4.99 million, and under 20 percent had expenditures of $5 million or more (it should be noted that 19 percent of health departments did not provide this information). Smaller health departments tended to spend more per person than larger ones ($48 for those serving fewer than 25,000 people versus $37 for those serving more than 1 million). Health departments governed by both state and local authorities reported higher median expenditures per person than those governed solely by state or local governments ($67 versus $46 and $38, respectively). This trend also pertains to local health department revenues. Smaller health departments reported median revenues of $54 per person, whereas median revenues for larger health departments were the same as median expenditures ($37 per person). Health departments operating under a shared governance model also experienced a higher median per capita than those governed solely by state or local governments ($67 versus $52 and $39, respectively), a trend that echoes local health department expenditures organized by these categories (NACCHO, 2011b).

Local health departments varied by population size in revenue sources as well. Federal direct and pass-though funds accounted for approximately 20 percent of revenues for local health departments serving fewer than 500,000 persons and for nearly 30 percent of those for departments serving populations of 500,000 or more. The percentage of revenues derived from Medicaid funding differed the most by population size. Larger local health departments serving more than 500,000 people received only 9 percent of their revenues from Medicaid, which accounted for more than 20 percent of revenues for those serving fewer than 25,000 people (NACCHO, 2011a). Many, regardless of size, received just less than 50 percent of their revenues from state and local sources.

## Workforce

The differences among local health departments are further exemplified by their workforces. While 87 percent of local health departments had fewer than 100 full-time employees in 2010, the median number ranged from 4 (for local health departments serving populations of fewer than 10,000) to 530 (for local health departments serving populations of 1 million or more). The percentage of full-time employees rose with the population size (73 percent for those serving populations of fewer than 10,000 to nearly 100 percent for those serving populations of 1 million or more). Most local health departments employed a range of personnel. Positions in at least 50 percent of local health departments included administrative personnel (97 percent), public health nurses and managers (96 and 85 percent, respectively), environmental health workers (81 percent), emergency preparedness staff (65 percent), health educators (57 percent), and nutritionists (55 percent). At the median, local health departments employed 17 full-time employees, 4 administrative or clerical personnel, 4 public health nurses, 2 environmental health workers, and 1 public health manager (NACCHO, 2011a).

## Role and Scope of Services

Local health departments provided a variety of services directly or through contracts with service providers in 2010 (NACCHO, 2011a). Local health departments offered the following 10 services most frequently: adult immunization, communicable disease surveillance, childhood immunization, tuberculosis screening, food service establishment inspection, environmental health surveillance, food safety education, tuberculosis treatment, school/child care facility inspection, and population-based nutrition services. Other common roles included monitoring and health surveillance, the development and enforcement of health policies and regulations, emergency response, communication of health issues, and mobilization of communities around important health issues (NACCHO, 2011a). Additional roles included serving as the source of primary and preventive care for a large portion of the uninsured population and Medicaid recipients, developing and training the county's health workforce, and linking the public to appropriate health services.

## Information Technology

Local health departments reported using information technology (IT) to varying degrees (NACCHO, 2011a). One issue of concern is interoperability with other IT systems. While 52 percent of local health departments could share some data, only 14 percent had IT systems that were fully compatible (NACCHO, 2010). Immunization registries were the most commonly used form of IT, followed by electronic health records, practice management systems, health information exchanges, and nationwide health information networks. Many local health departments reported using electronic syndromic surveillance systems for such activities as the detection of influenza-like and foodborne illnesses, the establishment of case definitions, and the evaluation of interventions (NACCHO, 2011a).

## REFERENCES

ASTHO (Association of State and Territorial Health Officials). 2011a. *ASTHO profile of state public health.* Arlington, VA: ASTHO.

ASTHO. 2011b. *Budget cuts continue to affect the health of Americans: Update May 2011.* Arlington, VA: ASTHO.

CMS Rural Health Center. 2011. *Medicare certified rural health clinics as of 7/12/2011.* https://www.cms.gov/MLNProducts/downloads/rhclistbyprovidername.pdf (accessed October 24, 2011).

HRSA (Health Resources and Services Administration). 2006. *Comparison of the rural health clinic and federally qualified health center programs.* Rockville, MD: HRSA.

HRSA. 2011a. *About the Ryan White HIV/AIDS Program.* http://hab.hrsa.gov/abouthab/aboutprogram.html (accessed November 15, 2011).

HRSA. 2011b. *Authorizing legislation: Section 330 of the Public Health Service Act (42 USC section 254b) authorizing legislation of the health center program.* http://bphc.hrsa.gov/policiesregulations/legislation/index.html (accessed January 4, 2012).

HRSA. 2011c. *Health center program terminology tip sheet.* http://bphc.hrsa.gov/technicalassistance /health_center_terminology_sheet.pdf (accessed January 19, 2012).

HRSA. 2011d. *HIV/AIDS program funding.* http://hab.hrsa.gov/data/reports/funding.html (accessed October 25, 2011).

HRSA. 2011d. *HIV/AIDS programs part A—grants to emerging metropolitan and transitional grant areas.* http://hab.hrsa.gov/abouthab/parta.html (accessed November 15, 2011).

HRSA. 2011f. *HIV/AIDS programs part B—grants to states and territories.* http://hab.hrsa.gov/abouthab/partbstates.html (accessed November 15, 2011).

HRSA. 2011g. *HIV/AIDS programs part C.* http://hab.hrsa.gov/abouthab/partc.html (accessed November 15, 2011).

HRSA. 2011h. *HIV/AIDS programs part D—services for women, infants, children, youth and their families.* http://hab.hrsa.gov/abouthab/partd.html (accessed November 15, 2011).

HRSA. 2011i. *HIV/AIDS programs SPNS—Special Projects of National Significance (part F).* http://hab.hrsa.gov/abouthab/partfspns.html (accessed November 15, 2011).

HRSA. 2011j. *Uniform Data System 2010 national data.* http://bphc.hrsa.gov/uds/view.aspx?year=2010 (accessed November 17, 2011).0

HRSA. 2011k. *What is a health center?* http://bphc.hrsa.gov/about/index.html (accessed October 24, 2011).

NACCHO (National Association of County and City Health Officials). 2005. *Operational definition of a functional local health department.* Washington, DC: NACCHO.

NACCHO. 2010. *The status of local health department informatics.* Washington, DC: NACHHO.

NACCHO. 2011a. *2010 national profile of local health departments.* Washington, DC: NACCHO.

NACCHO. 2011b. *Changes in size of local health department workforce.* Washington, DC: NACCHO.

National Association of Community Health Centers. 2011. Key health center data by state, 2010: National Association of Community Health Centers.

National Center for Farmworker Health. 2011a. *About community and migrant health centers.* http://www.ncfh.org/?sid=37 (accessed October 24, 2011).

National Center for Farmworker Health. 2011b. *Migrant health voucher programs.* http://www.ncfh.org/index.php?pid=65 (accessed October 24, 2011).

Novick, L. F., and G. P. Mays. 2005. *Public health administration: Principles for population-based management.* Sudbury, MA: Jones and Bartlett, Inc.

# Appendix C

# Meeting Agendas

The committee held data gathering sessions that were open to the public at four of its five general meetings and in three open sessions with CDC and HRSA. Five of these open meetings were held in Washington, DC; one in Irvine, California; and one in Denver, Colorado. The open session agendas for the public meetings are presented below.

## MEETING ONE

March 28, 2011
Keck Center of the National Academy of Sciences
500 Fifth Street, NW
Washington, DC 20001

1:00-2:30 PM        **Presentation of the Charge**
*Mary Wakefield, Ph.D., R.N.*
*Administrator*
*Health Resources and Services Administration*

*Judith A. Monroe, M.D.*
*Deputy Director, Centers for Disease Control and*
 *Prevention*
*Director, Office for State, Tribal, Local and*
 *Territorial Support*

*Chesley Richards, M.D., M.P.H., FACP*
*Director, Office of Prevention through Healthcare*
*Centers for Disease Control and Prevention*

**Committee Discussion**

2:30-5:00 PM          **Current Examples of Integration**
*Alina Alonso, M.D.*
*Director, Palm Beach County Health Department*
 *Florida Department of Health*

*Robert Resendes, M.B.A.*
*Health Officer/Director, Yavapai County*
 *Community Health Services, Arizona*

**Discussion**

*Ben Gramling*
*Director, Environmental Health Programs*
*Sixteenth Street Community Health Center,*
 *Milwaukee, Wisconsin*

*Charlie Alfero, M.A.*
*Chief Executive Officer, Hidalgo Medical Service,*
 *New Mexico*

**Discussion**

**MEETING TWO**

May 2, 2011
Keck Center of the National Academy of Sciences
500 Fifth Street, NW
Washington, DC 20001

9:30-10:30 AM          **Perspectives on Population Health**
*David B. Nash, M.D., M.B.A., FACP*
*Founding Dean, Jefferson School of*
 *Population Health*

*Helen Darling, M.A.*
*President and Chief Executive Officer, National*
 *Business Group on Health*

10:30-10:45 AM        **Break**

10:45 AM-12:00 PM     **Perspectives on Workforce**
                      *Barbara Safriet, J.D., L.L.M.*
                      *Visiting Professor of Law, Lewis & Clark*
                      *  Law School*

                      *Jean Johnson, Ph.D., FAAN*
                      *Dean and Professor, The George Washington*
                      *  University School of Nursing*

                      *Katherine Brieger, M.A., R.D., CDE*
                      *Chief Operating Officer, Hudson River*
                      *  Health Care*

12:00-1:00 PM         Lunch

1:00-2:30 PM          **Perspectives on Integration**
                      *M. Chris Gibbons, M.D., M.P.H.*
                      *Associate Director, Johns Hopkins Urban*
                      *  Health Institute*

                      *Ralph Fuccillo, M.A.*
                      *President, DentaQuest Foundation*

                      *Steven Woolf, M.D., M.P.H.*
                      *Director, Virginia Commonwealth University*
                      *  Center for Human Needs*


                      **MEETING THREE**

                      June 27, 2011
                 The Beckman Center, Newport Room
                      100 Academy Way
                      Irvine, CA 92617

9:30-10:30 AM         **Cardiovascular Disease**
                      *Michael Schooley, M.P.H.*
                      *Epidemiologist, Office on Smoking and Health*
                      *Centers for Disease Control and Prevention*

*Seiji Hayashi, M.D., M.P.H.*
*Chief Medical Officer, Bureau of Primary*
  *Health Care*
*Health Resources and Services Administration*

10:30-11:30 AM          **Colon Cancer Prevention and Screening**
*Marcus Plescia, M.D., M.P.H.*
*Director, Division of Cancer Prevention and*
  *Control*
*Centers for Disease Control and Prevention*

*Sarah Linde-Feucht, M.D.*
*Chief Public Health Officer*
*Health Resources and Services Administration*

*Natasha Coulouris, M.P.H.*
*Senior Public Health Advisor*
*Health Resources and Services Administration*

11:30 AM-12:30 PM       **Maternal and Child Health**
*Wanda Barfield, M.D., M.P.H.*
*Director, Division of Reproductive Health*
*Centers for Disease Control and Prevention*

*Chris DeGraw, M.D., M.P.H.*
*Senior Medical Advisor, Maternal and*
  *Child Health Bureau*
*Health Resources and Services Administration*

## MEETING FOUR

August 1, 2011
Keck Center of the National Academy of Sciences
500 Fifth Street, NW
Washington, DC 20001

10:00-11:00 AM          **HRSA Maternal and Child Health Bureau**
                        **Presentations**
                        **Overview**
*Chris DeGraw, M.D., M.P.H.*
*Senior Medical Advisor, Maternal and Child*
  *Health Bureau*

Title V of the Social Security Act Maternal and Child Health Infant Mortality Efforts
*Michele Lawler, M.S., R.D.*
*Deputy Director, Division of State and*
  *Community Health*

Secretary's Advisory Committee on Infant Mortality
*Beverly Wright, C.N.M., M.S.N., M.P.H.*
*Team Leader, Healthy Start Branch*
*Division of Healthy Start and Perinatal Services*

Maternal, Infant, and Early Childhood Home Visiting Program
*Audrey Yowell, Ph.D., M.S.S.S.*
*Chief, Policy, Program Planning and*
  *Coordination Branch*
*Division of Home Visiting and Early Childhood*
  *Systems*

Discussion

11:00 AM-12:00 PM CDC Maternal and Child Health Presentation
*Wanda Barfield, M.D., M.P.H., FAAP*
*Director, Division of Reproductive Health*
*National Center for Chronic Disease Prevention*
  *and Health Promotion*

Discussion

MEETING FIVE

August 2, 2011
Keck Center of the National Academy of Sciences
500 Fifth Street, NW
Washington, DC 20001

10:00-11:00 AM HRSA Cardiovascular Disease Presentations
*Natasha Coulouris, M.P.H.*
*Senior Public Health Advisor*

*Seiji Hayashi, M.D., M.P.H.*
*Chief Medical Officer, Bureau of Primary*
  *Health Care*

11:00 AM-12:00 PM   **CDC Cardiovascular Disease Presentations**
*Peter Briss, M.D., M.P.H.*
*Medical Director,*
*National Center for Chronic Disease*
  *Prevention and Health Promotion*

*Michael Schooley, M.P.H.*
*Epidemiologist, Office on Smoking and Health*

12:00-12:30 PM   **Lunch**

12:30-2:30 PM   **Discussion**


## MEETING SIX

August 11, 2011
Keck Center of the National Academy of Sciences
500 Fifth Street, NW
Washington, DC 20001

10:00-11:00 AM   **HRSA Colorectal Cancer Presentations**
*Matthew Burke, M.D.*
*Senior Clinical Advisor, Office of Quality and*
  *Data*
*Bureau of Primary Health Care*

*Suzanne Heurtin-Roberts, Ph.D., M.S.W.*
*Health Scientist, Office of Health Information*
  *Technology and Quality*

11:00 AM-12:00 PM   **CDC Colorectal Cancer Presentations**
*Marcus Plescia, M.D., M.P.H.*
*Director, Division of Cancer Prevention and*
  *Control*

12:00-12:30 PM   **Working Lunch**

12:30-2:30 PM   **Discussion**

## MEETING SEVEN

September 8-9, 2011
Inverness Hotel and Conference Center
200 Inverness Drive West
Englewood, CO 80112

8:30-10:00 AM
*Ellen-Marie Whelan, Ph.D., N.P., R.N.*
*Senior Advisor*
*CMS Innovation Center*

10:00-10:15 AM
*Reed Tuckson, M.D., FACP*
*Executive Vice President and Chief of*
*Medical Affairs*
*UnitedHealth Group*

# Appendix D

# Biosketches of Committee Members

**Paul J. Wallace, M.D.,** is director of the Center for Comparative Effectiveness Research at the Lewin Group. Formerly, Dr. Wallace was medical director of health and productivity management programs at the Permanente Federation. Dr. Wallace is an active participant, program leader, and perpetual student in clinical quality improvement, especially in the area of translation of evidence into care delivery using people- and technology-based innovation supported by performance measurement. As Kaiser Permanente's (KP's) medical director for health and productivity management programs, he led work to extend KP's experience with population-based care to further develop and integrate wellness, health maintenance, and productivity enhancement interventions. He also is active in the design and promotion of systematic approaches to comparative effectiveness assessment and accelerated organizational learning. Dr. Wallace was previously executive director of KP's Care Management Institute (CMI) from 2000 to 2005, and he continues as a senior advisor to CMI and to Avivia Health, the KP disease management company established in 2005. Dr. Wallace is a graduate of the University of Iowa School of Medicine and completed further training in internal medicine and hematology at Strong Memorial Hospital and the University of Rochester. Board-certified in internal medicine and hematology, he previously taught clinical and basic sciences and investigated bone marrow function as a faculty member at the Oregon Health Sciences University. Dr. Wallace is a member of the Board for AcademyHealth and serves as board chair for the Center for Information Therapy. He has previously served on the National Advisory Council for the Agency for Healthcare Research and Quality (AHRQ), the Medical

Coverage Advisory Committee for the Centers for Medicare & Medicaid Services, the Medical Advisory Panel for the Blue Cross and Blue Shield Technology Evaluation Center, the board of directors for DMAA: The Care Continuum Alliance, and the Committee on Performance Measurement and Standards Committee for the National Committee for Quality Assurance (NCQA). Dr. Wallace is a member of the Institute of Medicine (IOM) Board on Population Health and Public Health Practice and has participated in a number of IOM activities.

**Anne M. Barry, J.D., M.P.H.,** has 30 years of experience in state public service in a career that includes gubernatorial appointments to high-level leadership positions in four separate administrations. She currently serves as deputy commissioner for the Minnesota Department of Human Services, where she oversees both programmatic and operational activities. Immediately prior to her recent appointment as deputy commissioner in January 2011, Ms. Barry was chief compliance officer for the Department of Health and Human Services, with responsibility for legal, ethical, licensing, internal and external audit, and program oversight activities. Before joining the Department of Health and Human Services, Ms. Barry was appointed deputy commissioner of finance in the Governor Pawlenty administration after 4 years in that position for the Governor Ventura administration. As deputy commissioner of finance, she was responsible for overall agency leadership and management in the areas of accounting, budget, cash and debt management, economic forecasting, and financial information systems. Prior to her appointments in the Department of Finance, Ms. Barry was appointed by Governor Carlson as commissioner of health, a position she held from June 1995 to January 1999. She also served as deputy commissioner of health. Ms. Barry serves as adjunct faculty for the School of Public Health in the Academic Health Center at the University of Minnesota. She earned her juris doctorate from William Mitchell College of Law and her master of public health administration degree from the University of Minnesota. She also holds a bachelor of arts degree in occupational therapy from the College of St. Catherine. She is currently a candidate for a Ph.D. in kinesiology at the University of Minnesota.

**Jo Ivey Boufford, M.D.,** is president of the New York Academy of Medicine. Dr. Boufford also is professor of public service, health policy, and management at the Robert F. Wagner Graduate School of Public Service and clinical professor of pediatrics at New York University School of Medicine. She served as dean of the Robert F. Wagner Graduate School of Public Service at New York University from June 1997 to November 2002. Prior to that, she served as principal deputy assistant secretary for health in the Department of Health and Human Services (HHS) from November 1993 to January 1997, and as acting assistant secretary from January 1997 to May 1997. While at HHS, she served as U.S. representative on the executive board of the World Health Organization (WHO) from 1994 to 1997. From May 1991 to September 1993, Dr. Boufford served as director of the King's Fund College, London, England, a royal charity dedicated to the support of health and social services in London and the United Kingdom. She served as president of the New York City Health and Hospitals Corporation, the largest municipal system in the United States, from December 1985 until October 1989. Dr. Boufford was elected to membership in the IOM in 1992. She is currently the IOM foreign secretary and is a member of its Executive Council, Board on Global Health, and Board on African Science Academy Development. She attended Wellesley College for 2 years and received her B.A. (psychology) magna cum laude from the University of Michigan and her M.D., with distinction, from the University of Michigan Medical School. She is board-certified in pediatrics.

**Shaun Grannis, M.D., M.S., FAAFP,** is a research scientist with the Regenstrief Institute, Inc. and assistant professor of family medicine, Indiana University School of Medicine. He received an aerospace engineering degree from the Massachusetts Institute of Technology, and underwent postdoctoral training in medical informatics and clinical research at Regenstrief Institute and Indiana University School of Medicine. He joined Indiana University in 2001 and collaborates closely with national and international public health stakeholders to advance technical infrastructure and data sharing capabilities. Dr. Grannis is a member of WHO's Collaborating Center for the Design, Application, and Research of Medical Information Systems, where he provides consultancy on issues related to health information system identity management; the implementation of automated patient record matching strategies; and collaboration with WHO on the design, development, and implementation of enterprise medical record system architectures. Dr. Grannis recently completed an analysis of automated regional electronic laboratory reporting that revealed substantial increases in the electronic capture rates for diseases of public health significance as compared with traditional, manual, paper-based procedures. He developed methods for protecting the privacy and confidentiality of protected health information used for public health syndromic surveillance. He also is project director for an ongoing initiative integrating data flows from more than 120 hospitals across the state of Indiana for use in public health disease surveillance and clinical research. He serves as director of the Indiana Center of Excellence in Public Health Informatics. Dr. Grannis oversees the development of operational standards-based laboratory data interfaces between public health clinical laboratories and an electronic clinical messaging application used by both public health officials and clinicians.

As co-chair of the U.S. Health Information Technology Standards Panel's Population Health technical work group, he helped lead the development of technical interoperability specifications for nationally recognized public health information technology use cases.

**Larry A. Green, M.D.,** is professor and Epperson Zorn chair for innovation in family medicine and primary care at the University of Colorado School of Medicine. Previously, he practiced medicine in Van Buren, Arkansas, in the National Health Service Corps. He has remained a faculty member throughout his career, during which he has served in various roles, including practicing physician, residency program director, developer of practice-based research networks, and department chair. In 1999 he became founding director of the Robert Graham Center in Washington, DC, a research policy center sponsored by the American Academy of Family Physicians focused on family medicine and primary care. He served on the steering committee for the Future of Family Medicine Project, which advanced the development of the patient-centered medical home. He directed the Robert Wood Johnson Foundation's Prescription for Health national program, focused on incorporating health behavior change in redesigned primary care practices. He is a founding board member for Partnership 2040, a community-based participatory research enterprise in the Denver area. Dr. Green has received the Curtis Hames Award and the Maurice Wood Award for Lifetime Contribution to Primary Care Research. He is a member of the IOM. He graduated from Baylor College of Medicine in Houston, Texas, and performed his residency in family medicine in Rochester, New York, at Highland Hospital and the University of Rochester.

**Kevin Grumbach, M.D.,** is professor and chair of the Department of Family and Community Medicine at the University of California, San Francisco (UCSF). He is director of the UCSF Center for California Health Workforce Studies, co-director of the UCSF Center for Excellence in Primary Care, and co-director of the Community Engagement and Health Policy Program for the UCSF Clinical Translational Science Institute. His research interests include the health care workforce, innovations in the delivery of primary care, translational and implementation science, and racial and ethnic diversity in the health professions. With Tom Bodenheimer, he co-authored the best-selling textbook on health policy *Understanding Health Policy: A Clinical Approach* and the book *Improving Primary Care: Strategies and Tools for a Better Practice.* Dr. Grumbach received a Generalist Physician Faculty Scholar award from the Robert Wood Johnson Foundation, the Health Resources and Services Administration Award for Health Workforce Research on Diversity, and the Richard E. Cone Award for Excellence and Leadership in Cultivating Community Partnerships in Higher Education.

He is a member of the IOM. He practices family medicine at the Family Health Center at San Francisco General Hospital, and chairs the Primary Care Steering Committees for the San Francisco Department of Public Health and the UCSF Medical Center.

**Fernando A. Guerra, M.D., M.P.H.,** is director of health for the San Antonio Metropolitan Health District. Dr. Guerra's career reflects a long-standing interest and involvement in pediatric care, public health, and health policy. His expertise is in improving access to health care systems for infants, women, children, and the elderly and improving access to health care for migrant children. He is also active with local, national, and international forums on a variety of health issues. Dr. Guerra has served on the Committee on Ethical Issues in Housing-Related Health Hazard Research Involving Children; the Frontiers of Research on Children, Youth, and Families Steering Committee; the Committee on Using Performance Monitoring to Improve Community Health; and the Committee on Overcoming Barriers to Immunization. He is an IOM member and a former member of the Board on Children, Youth, and Families and has participated as a member of the Roundtable on Head Start Research. He has received the James Peavey Award from the Texas Public Health Association and the Job Lewis Smith Award from the American Academy of Pediatrics, and is a Kellogg Fellow of the Harvard School of Public Health, among many other awards and honors. Dr. Guerra holds a B.A. from the University of Texas at Austin, an M.P.H. from the Harvard School of Public Health, and an M.D. from the University of Texas Medical Branch at Galveston.

**James Hotz, M.D.,** is clinical services director and co-founder of Albany Area Primary Health Care, a community health center with 13 clinical sites that serves 40,000 citizens in rural Southwest Georgia. In addition to being a practicing internist, Dr. Hotz is heavily involved in health policy around issues of access and health disparity. He was a board member of the Georgia Association of Primary Health Care and was the first physician to be president of the association. Dr. Hotz served two terms on the board of the National Association of Community Health Centers (NACHC), is a member of the NACHC Clinical Services and Legislative Affairs Committees, and is coordinator for cancer screening for the NACHC Quality Center. Since 2006 Dr. Hotz has been on the Steering Committee of the Georgia State Cancer Plan and is co-chairperson of the Early Detection and Screening Work Group. He is medical director and serves on the board of directors of the Southwest Georgia Cancer Coalition, an organization that he helped found in 2001. Dr. Hotz is a member of the Council of Regional Cancer Coalitions of Georgia and was chairperson from 2004-2008. He is active in medical education, serving on the faculty of the Medical College of Georgia and the Admissions Committee of Mercer University School of Medicine. He is on the board of directors of the Southwest Georgia Area Health Education Center and was the founding president of the board in 1990. Dr. Hotz received the Clinical Recognition Award for Education and Training from NACHC in 1991, the Community Health Leadership Award from the Robert Wood Johnson Foundation in 1995, the Leadership Award of the Georgia Chapter of the American College of Physicians in 2008, and the James Alley Award for Outstanding Lifetime Achievement in Rural Health Care in 2009. In 2011 he was made a Master of the American College of Physicians. He is the author of the novel *Where Remedies Lie* based on his experience as a rural health center physician. A graduate of Cornell University and the Ohio State University School of Medicine, Dr. Hotz started his career as a legislative assistant to Kansas Representative Dr. William Roy addressing health reform issues.

**Alvin D. Jackson, M.D.,** is former director of the Ohio Department of Health. Previously he served as medical director of the Community Health Services Center in Fremont, Ohio; he began his career at the center during his 4-year family practice residency. During his tenure, the center expanded access to services with a fully equipped mobile unit, which extended health care services to 12 counties and has served as an immunization center at local schools. Dr. Jackson also served as chief of staff at Memorial Hospital in Fremont and staff physician at the Sandusky County Department of Health. He served as president of the Midwest Clinicians Network in 2000 and was clinician's state representative to the Ohio Association of Community Health Centers in 2001. Dr. Jackson has received Pfizer's Ohio Quality Care Award, HHS's Clinician Award, and a Robert Wood Johnson Community Health Leadership Award. He graduated from Andrew University in Michigan with a B.S. in biology, received his medical degree from the Ohio State University, and received an honorary doctor of humane letters degree from Heidelberg College.

**Bruce E. Landon, M.D., M.B.A., M.Sc.,** is professor of health care policy at Harvard Medical School and professor of medicine at the Beth Israel Deaconess Medical Center, where he practices internal medicine. Dr. Landon's primary research interest has been assessing the impact of different characteristics of physicians and health care organizations on physician behavior and the provision of health care services. He currently serves as principal investigator for an RO1 grant from the National Institute on Aging that involves studying the impact of physician financial incentives and other practice-related characteristics on the costs and intensity of care for Medicare beneficiaries. Dr. Landon has also been particularly interested in studying organizational approaches to improving the quality of care. He recently completed a national evaluation of the Health Resources and Services Administration (HRSA) Health Disparities Collaboratives, the primary quality improvement activity for the nation's community health centers. Dr. Landon has been interested in larger organizational entities, such as managed care health plans, as well, and has studied quality of care and patient experiences in Medicare's managed care program. He has extensively studied the experiences of state Medicaid agencies with managed care and compared quality within Medicaid managed care and private managed care plans. He also developed a research program with vascular surgeons to study the comparative effectiveness of treatment strategies for vascular disease. Dr. Landon graduated summa cum laude from the Wharton School at the University of Pennsylvania with a major in finance. He received his M.D. degree from the University of Pennsylvania School of Medicine and an M.B.A. with a concentration in health care management from the Wharton School. He also received an M.Sc. in health policy and management from the Harvard School of Public Health. Dr. Landon is a fellow of the American College of Physicians and an elected member of the American Society of Clinical Investigation.

**Danielle Laraque, M.D.,** is chair of the Department of Pediatrics and vice president of the Infants & Children's Hospital of Brooklyn, Maimonides Medical Center. Previously, she was chief of the Division of General Pediatrics and vice chair for public policy and advocacy at the Mount Sinai School of Medicine, Department of Pediatrics. Her academic appointments have included professor of pediatrics, professor of preventive medicine, and the Endowed Debra and Leon Black Professor of Pediatrics. Dr. Laraque received her B.S. in chemistry from the University of California, Los Angeles (UCLA). She completed her medical studies at UCLA, where she received the Roy Markus Scholarship. Her internship and residency were completed at the Children's Hospital of Philadelphia, where she was also a Robert Wood Johnson fellow in general academic pediatrics. Dr. Laraque directed the joint Mount Sinai Faculty Development Program for Primary Care and Clinician Research Fellowship (General Academic Pediatrics and General Internal Medicine), and over a period of about a decade trained countless fellows, residents, and medical students. She is a nationally and internationally recognized expert in injury prevention, child abuse, adolescent health risk behaviors, and health care delivery in underserved communities. In the past several years, she has focused on system changes to integrate the identification, diagnosis, and treatment of children's mental health problems in primary care settings. Dr. Laraque is immediate past president of the Academic Pediatric Association and was vice chair of the American Academy of Pediatrics (AAP) District II (New York State). She was AAP representative as the 2001 U.S. Public Health Service primary care policy fellow and was a member of the National Institute of Mental Health Standing Committee on Interventions for Disorders Involving Children and Their Families (2006-2010).

**Catherine G. McLaughlin, Ph.D.,** is a senior fellow at Mathematica Policy Research, Inc. (MPR). and professor in the Department of Health Management and Policy at the University of Michigan. Dr. McLaughlin has studied various topics related to health economics. She has published numerous articles on issues surrounding the working uninsured, the determinants of health plan choice, and market competition and health care costs. Her current research interests are focused on the impact of health information technology on health care markets, Medicare beneficiary enrollment behavior, patient-centered medical homes and low-income uninsured adults, disparities in health care utilization, and barriers to access. Dr. McLaughlin is an elected member of the IOM and the National Academy of Social Insurance and a member of the Council on Health Care Economics and Policy. She served as a senior associate editor of *Health Services Research* and is currently on its editorial board.

**J. Lloyd Michener, M.D.,** is professor and chairman of the Department of Community and Family Medicine at Duke University and director of the Duke Center for Community Research. He is a member of the board of the Association of Academic Medical Colleges, co-chair of the National Institutes of Health (NIH) Community Engagement Steering Committee, a member of the Centers for Disease Control and Prevention (CDC) Foundation Working Group on Public Health and Medical Education and the NIH Fogarty/Ellison Fellowship Program Selection Committee, and director of the Duke/CDC program in primary care and public health of the American Austrian Foundation Open Medical Institute. Dr. Michener is past president of the Association for Prevention Teaching and Research and past chair of the Council of Academic Societies of the Association of American Medical Colleges, and has served as a member of the board of the Association of Departments of Family Medicine and the National Patient Safety Foundation board of governers. He has played a leadership role in system redesign at Duke, including expansion of the physician assistant program and development of the master's program in clinical leadership. Dr. Michener has focused on finding ways of making health care work better through teams, community engagement, and practice redesign. He has overseen the obesity and chronic disease prevention programs of the Kate B. Reynolds Trust, a program designed to lower chronic disease rates in low-income areas across North Carolina, and the obesity prevention programs of the North Carolina Health and Wellness Trust Fund. Dr. Michener earned his undergraduate degree from Oberlin College in Ohio in 1974 and his medical degree from Harvard Medical School in 1978. He joined Duke as a resident in 1978, receiving the national Mead Johnson Award in Family Medicine in his senior year. He went on to become a Kellogg Fellow, after which he joined the Duke faculty in 1982.

**Robert L. Phillips, Jr., M.D., M.S.P.H.**, is a family physician and director of the Robert Graham Center: Policy Studies in Family Medicine and Primary Care in Washington, DC. The Graham Center functions as a division of the American Academy of Family Physicians, with editorial independence, staffed by a small research team focused on providing evidence to help inform policy making. It publishes extensively, most recently in the special primary care issue of *Health Affairs*, and was recently cited in both *Parade* magazine and *Forbes*. Dr. Phillips is a graduate of the University of Florida College of Medicine and underwent residency training at the University of Missouri, Columbia. He completed a 2-year National Research Service Award research fellowship and practiced in a federal housing federally qualified health center in Boone County, Missouri. He now practices part-time in a community-based residency program in Fairfax, Virginia. Dr. Phillips holds faculty appointments at Georgetown University, The George Washington University, and Virginia Commonwealth University. He recently served as vice chair of the U.S. Council on Graduate Medical Education, which advises the U.S. Congress and the administration.

**David N. Sundwall, M.D.**, is clinical professor of public health, University of Utah School of Medicine, and vice chair of the Medicaid and CHIP Payment and Access Commission (MACPAC). Dr. Sundwall served as executive director of the Utah State Department of Health from 2005 to 2010, where he supervised a workforce of more than 1,200 employees and a budget of almost $2 billion. He was president of the Association of State and Territorial Health Officials from 2007 to 2008. Dr. Sundwall served as president of the American Clinical Laboratory Association (ACLA) from September 1994 through May 2003, when he was appointed senior medical and scientific officer. The ACLA is a not-for-profit organization representing the leading national, regional, and local independent clinical laboratories. Previously, he was vice president and medical director of American Healthcare System (AmHS), at that time the largest coalition of not-for-profit multihospital systems in the country. Dr. Sundwall has extensive experience in federal government and national health policy, including service as administrator, HRSA, Public Health Service, HHS, and assistant surgeon general in the Commissioned Corps of the Public Health Service (1986-1988). During this period, he had adjunct responsibilities at HHS, including serving as co-chairman of the HHS Secretary's Task Force on Medical Liability and Malpractice and as the HHS Secretary's designee to the National Commission to Prevent Infant Mortality (1981-1986). Dr. Sundwall is board-certified in internal medicine and family practice and licensed to practice medicine in Utah and the District of Columbia.

**Mary Wellik, M.P.H., B.S.N.,** is former director of public health, Olmsted County, Minnesota, and has practiced public health in the community setting in clinic services and administration. Her practice has focused on strengthening community partnerships to improve health status and the development of public health policy. Ms. Wellik is past co-chair of the Minnesota eHealth Initiative and is a member of the National Association of County and City Health Officials Informatics work group. She has held numerous leadership positions, including in the local Community Healthcare Access Collaborative and in development of the Olmsted County Multicultural Healthcare Alliance. She served as co-chair of the Minnesota Health Improvement Partnership, member (current) of the governance board of the Southeast Minnesota Beacon Program, chair of the Local Public Health Association of Minnesota, and co-chair of its Legislative Committee.

**Winston F. Wong, M.D., M.S.,** serves as medical director for community benefit at Kaiser Permanente, with joint appointments at the Permanente Federation and the Kaiser Foundation Health Plan. In this role, he is responsible for developing and cultivating partnerships with communities and agencies in advancing population management and evidence-based medicine, with particular emphasis on safety net providers and the elimination of health disparities. Dr. Wong also is a member of multiple national advisory committees, addressing issues in cultural competence, health care access, and improving health care for vulnerable populations. A previous captain in the Commissioned Corp of the U.S. Public Health Service, Dr. Wong was awarded the Outstanding Service Medal while serving as both chief medical officer for HRSA, Region IX, and its director of California Operations. Dr. Wong received both his master's degree in health policy and his medical degree from the University of California, Berkeley-San Francisco Joint Medical Program. A board-certified family practitioner, he continues a practice in family medicine at Asian Health Services in Oakland, where he previously served as medical director. Dr. Wong also serves as vice chairperson for the National Council of Asian Pacific Islander Physicians.